A Health Information Book to
Answer Questions You Might Have
on Why There Should Be

DENTISTRY WITHOUT MERCURY

by
Sam Ziff
Michael F. Ziff, D.D.S.

-REVISED 2014 EDITION-
INCLUDING UPDATES FROM
THE INTERNATIONAL ACADEMY OF
ORAL MEDICINE & TOXICOLOGY
(IAOMT)
Compiled by Amanda R. Just

11th Revision and Update
Copyright © 1985-2014
By the International Academy of Oral Medicine and Toxicology and formerly by Bio-Probe, Inc.
All rights reserved

Printed in the USA
ISBN 978-0-9912986-0-0

Published by the International Academy of Oral Medicine and Toxicology (IAOMT)
8297 Champion'sGate Blvd. #193
Champion'sGate, FL 33896
Phone: (863) 420-6373   Fax: (863) 419-8136
Visit the IAOMT at http://www.iaomt.org

DEDICATION

To that small group of dentists, other health care providers, and researchers whose primary motivation has been to bring the scientific facts about the potential dangers of silver/mercury dental amalgam fillings to the attention of their patients and the public. They have persisted in the face of overwhelming peer and establishment pressures and unmitigated harassment. They have suffered the indignities of being called quacks and frauds in national media publications and have continued to practice mercury-free because their motivating force has always been the health and well-being of the patient.

This book is also dedicated to those tens of millions of unsuspecting and trusting dental patients who have had the poison mercury implanted in their teeth, under the name of "silver dental fillings" or "amalgam fillings" without their knowledge and/or consent. This poison has the potential to seriously impact their health, and it will continually escape from the fillings and accumulate in their bodies as long as the poison remains implanted in their teeth.

TABLE OF CONTENTS

2

WHO IS AT RISK FOR HEALTH COMPLICATIONS ASSOCIATED WITH DENTAL AMALGAM FILLINGS?
Pages 18-25

WHAT ARE THE SYMPTOMS OF MERCURY TOXICITY FROM DENTAL AMALGAM FILLINGS? *Pages 26-30*

WHAT ARE THE RESPONSIBILITIES OF THE UNITED STATES FOOD AND DRUG ADMINISTRATION (FDA) ON DENTAL AMALGAM FILLINGS? *Pages 30-34*

WHAT IS THE AMERICAN DENTAL ASSOCIATION (ADA) POSITION ON DENTAL AMALGAM FILLINGS?
Pages 35-41

WHAT ALTERNATIVES EXIST FOR TOOTH RESTORATIONS OTHER THAN DENTAL AMALGAM FILLINGS?
Pages 42-47

- Gold; *Pages 42-43*
- Composites (plastic resin fillings); *Pages 43-45*
- Glass Ionomer; *Page 45*
- Ceramic (porcelain); *Page 45-46*

WILL REPLACING DENTAL AMALGAM FILLINGS WITH ALTERNATIVE MATERIALS IMPROVE HEALTH?
Pages 47-50

IS REPLACING DENTAL AMALGAM FILLINGS DANGEROUS? *Pages 50-56*

- Safety measures during the amalgam removal procedure; *Pages 51-53*
- Dietary and nutritional safety measures; *Pages 53-54*
- Chelation; *Pages 54-55*
- Sweat therapy; *Pages 55-56*

HOW CAN I FIND OUT IF THE MERCURY COMING OUT OF MY DENTAL AMALGAM FILLINGS IS HURTING ME OR IF I AM HYPERSENSITIVE TO IT?
Pages 56-58

- Mercury exposure and mercury burden testing; *Pages 56-57*
- Mercury allergy and sensitivity testing; *Pages 57-58*
- Patient medical history; *Page 58*

4

For the purposes of this booklet, the number of scientific references was condensed. To research the detailed scientific evidence related to risks associated with dental amalgam mercury, visit the website of the International Academy of Oral Medicine and Toxicology at www.iaomt.org.

Also note that many revisions for the 2014 version of this booklet came from the following documents, both of which are available at www.iaomt.org with detailed scientific support:

Haley BE, Virtue WE. "Position statement of the International Academy of Oral Medicine and Toxicology in response to the 'Call for Information' extended by the Scientific Committee on Emerging and Newly Identified Health Risks (SCENIHR) European Commission." Champion'sGate, FL: IAOMT; October 10, 2012.

Kall JC, Robertson KM, Sukel PP, Just AR. "International Academy of Oral Medicine and Toxicology position statement against dental mercury amalgam fillings for medical and dental practitioners, dental students, and patients." Champion'sGate, FL: IAOMT; April 16, 2013.

WHAT IS MERCURY AND HOW TOXIC IS IT?

The element mercury is often called "quicksilver" due to its distinctive metallic color and its unique ability to rapidly move across surfaces. Similarly, its chemical symbol of "Hg" is based on the word "hydrargyrum," which means "water silver." Like gold, mercury occurs in natural deposits and cannot be created by humans.

Mercury exists in three major forms: 1) metallic mercury (used in thermometers, fluorescent bulbs, and amalgam fillings), 2) inorganic mercury compounds (used in batteries and certain beauty products), and 3) organic mercury (including methylmercury in fish and ethylmercury in vaccines).

The hazards of all types of mercury are recognized. For example, numerous state, national, and global environmental groups caution pregnant women and children against consuming seafood that might contain methylmercury. Additionally, authorities are working to reduce industrial mercury exposure from mercury-containing products such as thermometers, compact fluorescent light bulbs, batteries, electrical switches, and cosmetics, as well as mercury-releasing facilities such as crematoriums, coal-fired power plants, chloralkali factories, gold mining operatories, and dental offices.

While mercury has been used in medicine since ancient times, public awareness has grown during the past two centuries as a result of scientific studies and human tragedies that have repeatedly proven mercury poses significant risks to human health.

Based on such current evidence, a World Health Organization report warns of mercury:

> It may cause harmful effects to the nervous, digestive, respiratory, immune systems and to the kidneys, besides causing lung damage. Adverse health effects from mercury exposure can be: tremors, impaired vision and hearing, paralysis, insomnia, emotional instability, developmental deficits during fetal development, and attention deficit and developmental delays during childhood. Recent studies suggest that mercury may have no threshold below which some adverse effects do not occur.[1]

WHAT IS DENTAL AMALGAM?

Millions of dentists around the world routinely use dental amalgam as a filling material to repair decayed teeth. Often referred to as "silver" fillings, amalgam fillings actually consist of 45-55% metallic mercury.

Although mercury is the main ingredient, these dental restorations also contain different levels of copper, tin, silver, and zinc. Mercury, copper, and silver are all known to have toxic properties.

While there is clearly a lack of understanding among physicians, dentists, and patients about the health hazards of dental amalgam, there is likewise a lack of understanding about the dangers of mixing metals in the mouth.

If professionals and consumers understood these issues more clearly, many people might opt not to have amalgam fillings placed during dental procedures.

Thus, while mercury-containing restorations are commonly referred to as as "silver fillings," "dental amalgam," and/or "amalgam fillings," it would be more accurate to recognize them as "dental mercury amalgam fillings," "mercury silver fillings," or "mercury fillings."

Terminology recognizing the main ingredient of mercury is needed so that medical and dental practitioners, dental students, and patients are aware that mercury is the main ingredient in all dental amalgam fillings.

WHY HAVE DENTAL MERCURY AMALGAM FILLINGS BEEN USED FOR NEARLY 200 YEARS?

British chemist Joseph Bell is often credited with inventing mercury amalgam in 1812, but it was Auguste Taveau of France who produced the first dental amalgam by filing down silver coins and mixing the filed material with mercury to make a paste in 1816. The paste containing mercury, silver, and other metals undergoes a chemical reaction causing the material to harden after it has been placed into a cavity.

Discovering the ability of these metals to harden when placed in teeth was quite an innovation for the dental profession two centuries ago. It allowed greater numbers of people to be treated at less cost, since before the discovery of mercury fillings, the only options available were gold fillings or tooth extraction.

Consequently, mercury fillings catapulted dentistry from a cottage industry serving only those wealthy enough to afford gold fillings to the health industry of today which serves hundreds of millions of patients around the world.

Yet, controversy has surrounded the use of mercury in dentistry since the neurotoxin was first widely introduced as a filling material. The American Society of Dental Surgeons, the predecessor to the American Dental Association (ADA), made its members pledge not to use mercury because of its known toxicity,[2] and in more recent years, government officials, scientists, dentists, consumers, and many others have raised serious concerns about the threats dental mercury poses to humans and to the environment.

ARE DENTAL AMALGAM FILLINGS SAFE?

This question has been asked repeatedly for the nearly two centuries mercury has been used in dentistry. The fact that the question has been asked so many times sheds light on how debatable mercury fillings have been since their inception.

Mercury is a known poison. It is also very volatile. Specifically, "metallic" mercury gives off mercury vapor when agitated, compressed, or exposed to increases in temperature. If it is inhaled into the lungs, mercury vapor, which is colorless, tasteless, and odorless, can pass into the blood stream for distribution to all body tissues.

The governments of Norway, Sweden, and Denmark have banned the use of mercury amalgam fillings in dentistry, [3] [4] France has recommended that alternative mercury-free dental materials be used for pregnant women,[5] and Germany, Finland, Austria, and Canada have worked to reduce the use of dental mercury amalgam fillings for pregnant women, children, and patients with kidney problems.[6]

In 2013, over 90 countries signed the United Nations Environment Programme's Minamata Convention on Mercury, which is a global treaty that includes provisions aimed at minimizing the use of dental mercury and promoting cost-effective and clinically effective mercury-free alternatives for dental restorations.[7]

Some authorities in the United States have also recognized the dangers of mercury from dental amalgam fillings, and brochures have been created to educate patients about their choices for tooth restorations in California,[8] Connecticut,[9] Maine,[10] and Vermont.[11] The brochures, which are required to be presented to dental patients, contain information about the release of mercury vapor from dental mercury amalgam fillings and concerns related to amalgam usage, as well as information about mercury pollution to the environment caused by dental mercury.

Yet, dentists in the United States, largely encouraged by the American Dental Association (ADA), have been taught to believe that once mercury has been mixed into the filling material, it remains "locked in" and cannot be released.

Unfortunately, this is not the case, and research continues to show that mercury leaches out of amalgam fillings. To illustrate this hazard, scientific evidence published in 2011 demonstrates that more than 67 million Americans aged two years and older exceed the intake of mercury vapor considered "safe" by the U.S. Environmental Protection Agency (EPA) due to the presence of dental mercury amalgam fillings, whereas over 122 million Americans exceed the intake of mercury vapor considered "safe" by the California EPA due to their dental mercury amalgam fillings.[12]

Likewise, research clearly demonstrates that dental amalgam exposes dental professionals, dental staff, and dental patients to mercury vapor (gaseous releases of mercury), mercury-containing particulate (solid releases of mercury), and other forms of mercury contamination.[13 14 15 16 17 18 19 20 21 22]

WHAT CAUSES THE MERCURY TO ESCAPE FROM A DENTAL AMALGAM FILLING?

A variety of scenarios can cause mercury to be emitted from amalgam fillings, and these include stimulated releases and unstimulated releases, as well as corrosion of the tooth restoration. Each of these occurrences is described in more detail here:

Release of mercury from dental amalgam with stimulation

Certain situations can provoke higher levels of mercury to be emitted from amalgam fillings. Basically, when mercury is heated up, more vapor is released due to the increase in temperature, which can obviously occur due to friction from teeth rubbing together or the use of a dental instrument on the filling.

Therefore, it makes logical sense that studies have shown mercury vapor is released from dental amalgam fillings at higher rates during chewing, brushing, cleaning, clenching of teeth, etc., [23] [24] [25] [26] [27] and that mercury is released during the placement, replacement, and removal of dental amalgam fillings. [28] [29] [30] [31]

Release of mercury from dental amalgam without stimulation

For many years, very little scientific consideration was given to the non-stimulated release of mercury from amalgam fillings because all of the attention had been focused on the amount of mercury vapor released by chewing, brushing, grinding, dental work, and other provocations.

However, in 1987 researchers in Sweden concluded that the continual release of mercury vapor from amalgam fillings (which occurs regularly for 24 hours a day and 365 days a year) is a major contributor to total mercury body burden. [32] This basically established that mercury escapes from the fillings all the time.

Indeed, recent data has shown that an individual accumulates a constant dose of mercury throughout the lifetime of a dental mercury amalgam filling. [33]

Equally troubling is that once inside the mouth, mercury remains a retained heavy metal until the body can excrete the toxin.[34]

Release of mercury in saliva from amalgam fillings

Research has demonstrated that mercury is discharged into saliva[35] and the body uptake from swallowed mercury can be significant for individuals with a large number of amalgam fillings.[36] [37]

The important point to remember is that mercury vapor, ions, and abraded particles are escaping and being inhaled, swallowed, and absorbed by the oral and nasal mucosa continuously during the lifetime of an amalgam filling.[38]

Release of mercury due to corrosion of amalgam fillings

Another phenomenon that occurs in the mouth can also contribute to the release of mercury, and it is called corrosion. Corrosion is similar to "rust" and means that surface particles of the filling material are chemically broken down and released into the oral cavity.

Thus, while mercury vapor is released during chewing or grinding, miniscule "rusted" particles of amalgam are also being eroded, taken into food or saliva, and swallowed.

Concerns have been raised that these small mercury-containing particles can be triggered to produce methylmercury inside the human body. Bacteria in soil and water can convert mercury into methylmercury, a form of the element sometimes consumed by fish and shellfish,[39] and due to serious health risks, pregnant women and children are advised not to eat seafood that might contain methylmercury.[40]

Understanding the process of how methylmercury is created has led to research exploring the ability of metallic mercury rooted in the human system (such as that from amalgam fillings) to be transformed into methylmercury in the mouth[41] [42] [43] [44] and by specific strains of yeast and bacteria that dwell in the gut.[45] [46]

Another disturbing discovery is that mercury from amalgam dental fillings can cause gingival and intestinal microflora to become mercury resistant and antibiotic resistant.[47]

More about corrosion and oral galvanism

When exposed to moisture and oxygen, amalgam will corrode or oxidize like most other metals. This is comparable to a car battery, which has two or more dissimilar metals suspended in an acid solution. In a car battery, the corrosion of the metals results in the production of electrical currents.

Similarly, in a human mouth, amalgam fillings, which normally contain three or four different types of metals, interact with saliva. The saliva provides the electrolyte because it contains various elements such as calcium, magnesium, and potassium, in addition to acid.

So, the mouth with an amalgam filling has all the necessary ingredients available to create electrical currents, and these electrical currents can even be measured. This phenomenon is called "oral galvanism," and it literally means that the oral cavity is like a small car battery or miniature electrical generator.

When a person's "mouth battery" starts generating electrical currents, the corrosion of the amalgam fillings is intensified. This increases both the amount of mercury vapor and the amount of broken off particles that can be released into the oral cavity.[48] It can also be instrumental in the release of free mercury droplets from the filling.[49]

Furthermore, electrolytic corrosion can be enhanced by gold and mercury fillings being in contact with each other. Namely, if there is an amalgam filling under a gold crown or if a gold filling or crown is in contact with an opposing or adjacent amalgam filling, it can exacerbate corrosion and increase the release of mercury particles and vapor into the oral cavity. Even standard dental textbooks have warned against this for years.[50]

A new area of consideration is also the potential for dental amalgam fillings to react with titanium implants, and researchers have warned that the combination of these metals can result in systemic dermatitis.[51]

Overall, it is essential to understand that dissimilar metals in the mouth can contribute to electrical activity and corrosion and that in some individuals, this can cause unexplained pain, ulcerations, inflammation, and other conditions.[52]

WHO IS AT RISK FOR HEALTH COMPLICATIONS ASSOCIATED WITH DENTAL AMALGAM FILLINGS?

Unfortunately, the mercury in amalgam fillings can harm anyone who has them in their mouth, anyone who works with dental amalgam as part of their occupation, as well as the children of mothers with these fillings and the children of mothers who work with dental amalgam. Additionally, certain conditions can intensify a person's negative reaction to mercury. Each of these groups is described on the next several pages:

The general population

Mercury vapor is continuously emitted from dental mercury amalgam fillings, and particulate can also be discharged from dental mercury amalgam fillings, which means that all dental patients who have amalgam fillings are directly exposed to mercury.[53] [54]

The output of mercury is intensified by the number of fillings present and other

18

activities such as chewing, teeth-grinding, brushing, dental treatments and procedures, and even the consumption of hot liquids.[55] [56] [57] [58] This includes mercury released during hygiene, cleaning, and polishing procedures, and mercury released during placement of new restorations and removal of old ones.

What this means is that all dental patients are potentially at risk from mercury released from their amalgam fillings. Yet, each patient is unique, and a variety of other circumstances can influence the level of harm from the fillings.

Pregnant women and children

In 2009, 19 members of the U.S. Congress wrote a letter to the U.S. Food and Drug Administration (FDA) to express their concern about mercury used in amalgam fillings with a focus on potential dangers to pregnant women and children.[59]

Prior to that, when Representative Diane Watson of California introduced the *Mercury Filling Disclosure and Prohibition Act* (H.R. 2101), she explained, "It is, in fact, children who are at greatest risk from these fillings."[60]

Many others have likewise recognized that the well-being of pregnant women and children is jeopardized by the use of amalgam fillings, and studies confirm that fetal and infant exposure to mercury via maternal dental amalgam can have health consequences.[61] [62] [63] [64] [65]

Another reason for grave concern is that mercury is excreted in breast milk of mothers with dental mercury amalgam fillings, and the mercury concentration in breast milk increases as the number of amalgam fillings in the mother increases.[66] [67]

Specifically, a study published in 2011 noted, "As we showed, the number of amalgam filled teeth in breast-feeding mothers strongly influences the mercury level in their milk. Take it into consideration that maternal milk is the only source of nutrition during the first few months after birth…"[68]

Research also demonstrates that children are at-risk for health impairments caused by dental amalgam mercury fillings.[69] [70] [71]

In fact, a 2011 study cautioned, "Changes in dental practices involving amalgam, especially for children, are highly recommended in order to avoid unnecessary exposure to Hg [mercury]."[72]

On another note, in 2012, an official "Crimes against Humanity" complaint was filed with the International Criminal Court (ICC) at The Hague against those involved in an $11 million experiment conducted on children to test the safety of dental amalgam. The studies, collectively known as the "Children's Amalgam Trials" (CAT),[73] [74] were funded by the U.S. government's National Institute of Dental and Cranial Research (NIDCR).

The CAT mercury experiments were administered on children aged 8-10 from low income families in New England and at the Casa Pia orphanage in Lisbon from 1997-2005. Even when personnel at Casa Pia were convicted of running a large pedophile ring abusing the children in 2002,[75] the study continued.

The late Sandra Duffy, a lawyer from Oregon, noted in 2004 that the U.S. consent forms given to parents in New England did "not disclose how much mercury exposure or absorption occurs from the fillings," and the Portuguese consent forms, 100 of which were signed by the same doctor, did not even disclose that the fillings contained mercury.[76]

Although many have used the controversial results of the CAT experiments to suggest that using amalgam is safe for children, other evidence has shown the contrary. Boyd Haley, PhD, found major scientific flaws in the original CAT study design, [77] and in 2010, David and Mark Geier, MD, published an assessment of the Casa Pia Children's Amalgam Trial which revealed that the original children's study did not account for the chronic exposure that would occur as a result of amalgam fillings being in the subjects' mouth for many years of their lives.[78]

Perhaps the hazard of using dental mercury in children was best acknowledged at a 2010 FDA Dental Products Panel when Dr. Suresh Kotagal, a pediatric neurologist at the

Mayo Clinic, concluded, "...I think that there is really no place for mercury in children."[79]

It is not surprising that some countries have already placed restrictions on the use of dental amalgam for pregnant women and children.[80]

Dental workers, dental school students, and visitors to the dental office

Dentists, dental staff, and dental students are exposed to mercury at a greater rate than their patients because they routinely work with amalgam fillings. For this reason, it is not surprising that research has demonstrated the presence of dangerous levels of mercury in the dental workplace.[81] [82]

Scientific data also indicates that the reproductive systems of female dental personnel are potentially impacted by occupational exposure to mercury.[83] One study, which was conducted at the National Institute of Environmental Health Sciences, determined that there was reduced fertility among dental assistants with occupational exposure to mercury.[84]

Another outcome of the use of mercury in dentistry is the chronic exposure to individuals in any and all areas of the dental office. Severe exposures from past practices in dental offices included the hand-squeezing of fresh amalgam, where drops of liquid mercury could run over the dentist's hands and contaminate the entire office.[85]

The concept that dental work areas are home to a plethora of toxic mercury exposures is one that requires far more consideration as far as changes in practices necessary to protect dental workers and visitors to the office.

Individuals who are allergic to mercury

The issue of individuals being unaware of conditions that can impact their reaction to amalgam fillings also applies to allergies. Allergy to mercury is a completely separate health issue from toxicity, but it merits equal attention because approximately 21 million American are estimated to be allergic to mercury.[86]

This suggests that while most doctors do not test their patients for mercury allergy, some patients are allergic or sensitive to the dental mercury amalgam fillings in their mouths.[87][88][89][90][91][92]

People can also develop mercury allergies after the fillings are placed, and interestingly enough, research suggests mercury allergies are more likely to develop after expsoure to the metal has occurred. To illustrate this point, data has established that exposure to dental mercury amalgam fillings correlates with a higher prevalence of mercury allergies.[93]

Individuals with a genetic predisposition to mercury illness

One area of mercury science that is rapidly growing involves recognition that individuals with certain genetic characteristics cannot endure exposure or excrete mercury from their bodies as well as others. For instance, research has established that mercury exposure from dental amalgam particularly threatens individuals with genetic variants such as CPOX4, APOE(3,4), and BDNF polymorphisms.[94][95][96]

Additionally, recent research has identified a genetic predisposition to neurological impacts by mercury exposure from dental amalgam in certain male children.[97]

Another study suggests that roughly 25% of the U.S. population is polymorphic for a specific genetic trait associated with sensitivity to mercury toxicity,[98] which amounts to 78 million Americans today.

Since most people are unaware of their genetic circumstances, it is not possible to warn individuals about this issue.

Individuals with conditions potentially caused or worsened by exposure to mercury

Whereas some groups have attempted to deny that amalgam fillings can cause serious health issues, numerous studies show otherwise. A variety of ailments are known to be caused or worsened by toxic exposures. Obviously, any toxic exposure burdens the human body and impairs its ability to fight off other illnesses.

That being said, the mercury in dental amalgam fillings can potentially exacerbate and contribute to all of the conditions stated below, as well as a myriad of other health problems:

- Alzheimer's disease[99]
- Amyotrophic Lateral Sclerosis (Lou Gehrig's disease)[100]
- Antibiotic resistance[101]
- Autism Spectrum Disorders [102] [103] [104]
- Autoimmunity /Immune dysfunction/ Immunodeficiency[105] [106] [107]
- Cardiovascular problems[108]
- Chronic Fatigue Syndrome[109] [110] [111]
- Complaints of unclear causation[112] [113] [114] [115]
- Hearing loss[116]
- Kidney problems[117] [118] [119] [120]
- Micromercurialism[121]
- Multiple sclerosis [122] [123] [124]
- Oral lichenoid reaction [125] [126] [127] [128] [129] [130] and oral lichen planus[131] [132]
- Parkinson's disease[133]
- Periodontal disease[134] [135]
- Reproductive dysfunction[136] [137]
- Symptoms of chronic mercury poisoning[138]

25

WHAT ARE THE SYMPTOMS OF MERCURY TOXICITY FROM DENTAL AMALGAM FILLINGS?

Categorizing the potential symptoms attributed to mercury exposure from fillings is a complex matter. To put it simply, each person's symptoms are based on the individual's body, and therefore, ailments related to mercury manifest themselves in a large variety of ways.

While this "one size does not fit all" description of mercury-related illness is confusing, it does help to explain why two individuals with amalgam fillings can react to them completely differently.

Basically, mercury has the ability to act like a chameleon, camouflaging a different set of problems within each human body environment. This is because there are countless factors that dictate a person's reaction to mercury. For example, in addition to the situations outlined in the previous section of this booklet, selenium levels,[139] exposure to lead,[140] [141] [142] [143] and consumption of milk[144] [145] or alcohol,[146] can also play a role in each person's unique response to mercury.

Thus, mercury-related symptoms are quite diverse and independent to each individual. With that in mind, the information below provides generalized lists of symptoms[147] [148] [149] for patients, professionals, and parents to review when evaluating potential ailments related to the mercury in amalgam fillings:

ELEMENTAL MERCURY EXPOSURE

1. PSYCHOLOGICAL DISTURBANCES

Irritability

Shyness or timidity

Lack of attention

Loss of self-confidence

Decline of intellect

Lack of self-control

Insomnia

Nervousness

Loss of memory

Fits of anger

Depression

Anxiety

Drowsiness

2. ORAL CAVITY DISORDERS

Bleeding gums

Loosening of teeth

Foul breath

Alveolar bone loss

Excessive salivation

Metallic taste

Leukoplakia (white patches)

Gingivitis (inflammation of the gums)

Stomatitis (mouth inflammation)

Ulceration of gingiva, palate, tongue

Burning sensation in mouth or throat

Tissue pigmentation

3. GASTROINTESTINAL EFFECTS

Abdominal cramps

Constipation or diarrhea

Gastrointestinal problems including colitis

4. SYSTEMIC EFFECTS

CARDIOVASCULAR: Irregular heartbeat (tachycardia, bradycardia); Feeble and irregular pulse; Alterations in blood pressure; Chest pain

NEUROLOGICAL: Chronic or frequent headaches; Dizziness; Ringing or noises in ears; Fine tremors (hands, feet, lips, eyelids, tongue)

RESPIRATORY: Persistent cough; Emphysema; Shallow and irregular respiration

IMMUNOLOGICAL: Allergies; Asthma; Rhinitis (inflammation of the nose); Sinusitis; Lymphadenopathy, especially cervical (neck)

ENDOCRINE: Subnormal temperature; Cold, clammy skin, especially hands and feet; Excessive perspiration

OTHER: Muscle weakness; Speech disorders; Dim or double vision; Fatigue; Hypoxia (lack of oxygen); Anemia; Edema (swelling); Loss of weight; Loss of appetite (anorexia); Joint pains

5. SEVERE CASES
Hallucinations   Manic depression
Suicidality

ORGANIC MERCURY EXPOSURE

1. EARLIEST SYMPTOMS

Fatigue

Headache

Inability to concentrate

Forgetfulness

Outbursts of anger

Depression

Decline of intellect

Apathy

2. PROGRESSED SYMPTOMS

Numbness and tingling of hands, feet, lips

Muscle weakness progressing to paralysis

Dim or restricted vision

Hearing difficulty

Speech disorders

Loss of memory

Lack of coordination

Emotional instability

Dermatitis

Renal damage (kidney)

General central nervous system dysfunctions

The study of micromercurialism (low level exposure to mercury) suggests that continual exposure to small doses of mercury over long periods of time (such as from dental amalgam) can produce many of the symptoms listed in the preceding pages.

Additionally, mercury is so toxic to the human organism that there can be cell death or irreversible chemical damage long before clinically observable symptoms indicate that something is wrong. In fact, mercury in the brain has a half life of over 20 years.[150] This means that it takes more than 20 years to get rid of 1/2 of a single dose of mercury in the brain. Due to this long half life, it makes sense that it is only a matter of time and degree of mercury exposure until some form of symptomatology appears.

Unfortunately, since mercury exposure from dental amalgam can be prolonged and the onset of the symptoms can vary so dramatically, they may not be associated with dental mercury. This is especially true because most people do not have all of their fillings put in at the same time, which means symptoms from amalgam mercury exposure can gradually manifest themselves over the course of many years.

WHAT ARE THE RESPONSIBILITIES OF THE UNITED STATES FOOD AND DRUG ADMINISTRATION (FDA) ON DENTAL AMALGAM FILLINGS?

By law, the Food and Drug Administration (FDA) is required to classify all medical devices (including dental devices) accepted for use in the United States. If a material is not classified, it cannot be considered an approved device. Taking this into account, this section outlines the history of the FDA's difficulty with classifying amalgam fillings.

Regulatory issues with dental amalgam were immediately obvious when the "Medical

Device Amendments Act" was passed by Congress in 1976. This amendment created the requirement for the FDA to categorize all medical devices.[151]   At that time, the commissioner announced that mercury fillings would be considered "implants," which require more stringent evaluation than other medical devices because they are placed in the human body.   Although the American Dental Association (ADA) asked for dental amalgam to be exempt from the rule, the commissioner denied the request.

In 1980, the FDA published a report with suggestions about how to classify various dental devices, including those containing mercury.[152]   Over the next few years, the FDA succeeded in categorizing all dental filling materials except for mercury amalgam.

When the Final Rule of the FDA on Classifications of Dental Devices was published in the Federal Register on August 12, 1987,[153] there was no mention or classification of dental amalgam as a dental device.   Instead, the individual components of amalgam were approved and classified: Mercury was placed in Class I (less risk, no proof of safety needed), and amalgam alloy (the material mixed with the mercury to form amalgam) was placed in Class II (more risk, no proof of safety needed).   The rationale behind not classifying dental amalgam in its finished form was due to the suggestion that amalgam be considered a "reaction product" prepared in the dental office, thereby not permitting authorities to review the actual final product. However, this was a clear violation of the intent of Congress and the Medical Device Amendment, which requires proof of safety for devices implanted into the human body.

In essence, the attempts not to classify these fillings can be seen as a maneuver to circumvent identifying dental amalgam as an implant. The attempts can also be seen as a means to avoid classifying the final product by classifying each ingredient separately instead.

It is especially concerning because the manufacturer provides the components of dental amalgam in a single capsule separated only by a membrane. The amalgam manufacturer also determines how much mercury is placed in the capsule and the metallic content (formula) of the alloy placed in the capsule. The dentist and/or dental staff follow the manufacturer's instructions, and dental workers have absolutely no control over determining how much mercury is eventually placed into the mouth of the patient.

Meanwhile, in 1988, the FDA ruled that mercury and its compounds are NOT "Generally Recognized as Safe" (GRAS) and eliminated mercury from products sold "over-the-counter" (OTC).[154]

So, whereas mercury products were removed from sale in over-the-counter products, the FDA continued to allow mercury-containing dental amalgam to be placed into people's teeth.

Several years later, however, a Dental Products Panel of the FDA convened on March 15, 1991, to consider the issue of amalgam fillings. Lars Friberg, MD, PhD, of the Karolinska Institute, Stockholm, Sweden, and Alfred Zamm, MD, warned that amalgam fillings were both dangerous and unfit for human use.

In spite of the meeting, no official classification of dental amalgam (as a finished product) was offered by the FDA. However, finally in 2002, the FDA announced its failure to classify dental amalgam over the years was "inadvertent," although they eventually rescinded that statement.[155] Later in 2002, the American Dental Association (ADA) and FDA succeeded in allowing amalgams to be used without a proof of safety.

Due to many comments and complaints as a result of that 2002 ruling, the FDA invited experts to provide scientific data with regards to the health risks of mercury amalgam in September of 2006. Two scientific advisory committees voted that the FDA was mistaken in deeming mercury fillings as safe, and an advisory panel voted down a "White Paper" presented by the FDA about amalgam fillings. (A "White Paper" is a government document written to explain a policy, and it often serves as a precursor to legislation.) In the end, yet again, no official classification of the finished product was issued.[156]

On December 28, 2007, *Moms against Mercury* filed a lawsuit alleging that the FDA had willfully avoided classifying dental amalgam. By June of 2008, the case was settled, and the FDA agreed to classify dental amalgam within thirteen months.[157]

On July 28, 2009, the FDA announced that it was classifying dental mercury amalgam in Class II, thus not requiring proof of safety.[158] FDA's Final Rule on this issue was published,[159] and subsequently, the FDA also published an Addendum in support of its Final Rule.[160] An FDA warning for dental amalgam mercury use in developing children and fetuses posted one year earlier[161] was then removed from the FDA website in 2009.

The IAOMT sponsored a Petition for Reconsideration later that year which identified errors made by the FDA.[162] Based on the IAOMT petition, the FDA scheduled a meeting of the Dental Products Panel of the Medical Devices Advisory Committee in December 2010. At the meeting, the Dental Products Panel encouraged the FDA to consider limiting dental mercury amalgam use in pregnant women and children and to consider labeling that would warn consumers about the risks of this mercury-containing product.[163]

A decision on the issue was expected from the FDA by December 31, 2011,[164] but as of this book's publication, no decision about dental amalgam fillings based on these remaining controversies has been issued.

WHAT IS THE AMERICAN DENTAL ASSOCIATION (ADA) POSITION ON DENTAL AMALGAM FILLINGS?

First of all, many people are confused as to what the American Dental Association (ADA) actually is. It is *not* a government authority, nor is it a medical research organization. Rather, the ADA is a professional trade group of dentists, who are invited to join and pay dues to the association.

The American Society of Dental Surgeons, the predecessor to the ADA, made its members pledge not to use mercury because of its known toxicity.[165] However, due to arguments about using amalgam in dentistry, the group collapsed in 1856. Shortly thereafter, the ADA was founded with the premise that putting toxic mercury in the mouths of dental patients via amalgam fillings was an acceptable practice.

The ADA has stuck to its pro-amalgam position for the past century and a half, and the decision has been lucrative since inexpensive mercury-containing fillings vastly expanded the business of dentistry.

However, the ADA's defense has faltered in more recent years. The first notable example of this occurred in July of 1984, when the National Institute of Dental Research (NIDR) sponsored a "Workshop on the Biocompatibility of Metals in Dentistry" hosted by the ADA. After this workshop, the ADA officially acknowledged that mercury is released from amalgam fillings, although they went on to state that the amount released is so small that it could not cause any health problems except in those individuals who might be hypersensitive or allergic to mercury.[166]

The ADA continued to suggest amalgam fillings were safe, but the shaky basis for their position was made gruesomely apparent by a 1990 position paper in the *Journal of the American Dental Association* which identified the main source for the ADA's defense of mercury fillings:

> The strongest and most convincing support we have for the safety of dental amalgam is the fact that each year more than 100 million amalgam fillings are placed in the United States. And since amalgam has been used for more than 150 years, literally billions of amalgam fillings have been successfully used to restore decayed teeth.[167]

Think about that! The ADA provided the weakest example of "anecdotal" evidence possible as their scientific proof that amalgam fillings were safe. What they were really saying was that they had absolutely no convincing scientific evidence proving that the mercury released from amalgam fillings was not causing mercury poisoning.

Yet, the ADA must have been terribly concerned about the tenuous legal nature of their position on the safety of amalgam. Otherwise, there could not possibly be any rational reason for their creation of a "gag order" that prohibits dentists from suggesting the removal of dental amalgam as a means of lowering toxic exposure.

To be precise, the ADA's updated code of ethics explains "removal of amalgam restorations from the non-allergic patient solely for the alleged purpose of removing toxic substances from the body, when such treatment is performed at the recommendation or suggestion of the dentist, is improper and unethical."[168]

This clause remains intact today, so while it is perfectly legal and acceptable for a patient to request removal of their amalgam restorations, a dentist is not supposed to recommend removal as a means to reduce toxic levels in the body.

Unfortunately, a number of dentists have faced reprimand and humiliation for violating the ADA gag order, and cases of dentists having to fight this rule have actually gone to court.[169] While dentists have been known to turn each other in for violating this order, the ADA has also gone so far as to file complaints themselves. Such was the case in the 1995 trial of Dr. Hal Huggins who lost his dental license but has since continued to educate people around the world about illnesses related to dangerous dental practices.

When the tables were turned in a 1995 civil lawsuit filed against the ADA over amalgam fillings, the ADA abandoned its frequently stated obligation to support practicing dentists and the best interests of public health and adroitly absolved itself of any responsibility. In fact, in a legal brief filed with the court for that case, attorneys for the ADA made the following argument:

> The ADA owes no legal duty of care to protect the public from allegedly dangerous products used by dentists. The ADA did not manufacture, design, supply or install the mercury-containing amalgams. The ADA does not control those who do. The ADA's only alleged involvement in the product was to provide information regarding its use. Dissemination of information relating to the practice of dentistry does not create a duty of care to protect the public from potential injury.[170]

The Court agreed with the ADA and dismissed it from the case. This information should send chills down the spines of amalgam-using dentists and amalgam-bearing consumers.

Speaking of consumers, it is quite interesting that the ADA, while washing its hands of protecting the public in the 1995 civil lawsuit, has been offering a Seal of Acceptance program for dental products since 1930.[171] A 1999 article in the *LA Times* noted that amalgam consumer products are endorsed by the ADA and that some dentists "think the ADA is biased because it is paid for the endorsements."[172]

Another issue that raises red flags is the ADA's public relations campaigns against any mainstream media event that presents evidence contrary to their defense of dental amalgam.

In December 1990, CBS television aired an episode of *60 Minutes* featuring a segment entitled "Is There Poison in Your Mouth?"[173] In it, Morley Safer addressed ADA spokespersons as to why dentists would be attacked for removing amalgam fillings due to concerns about health. The ADA representatives appeared to be uncomfortable during the show, and the ADA launched a massive damage control campaign after the show aired.

An article by Keith W. Sehnert, MD, Gary Jacobson, DDS, and Kip Sullivan, JD, described the aftermath of the *60 Minutes* segment:

> The dental establishment was furious with CBS. The ADA attacked CBS in the January 7, 1991 edition of its newspaper for 'the irresponsible ways in which

viewers were led to the conclusion that amalgam fillings are unsafe.' To the contrary, said the ADA, 'scientific evidence suggests mercury amalgam is safe to use.' The ADA newspaper published statements by Dr. Harold Loe, director of National Institute of Dental Research, criticizing CBS for having 'an obvious bias' against amalgams. Dentists all over the country received information packets from the ADA, including copies of the ADA newspaper and a 1986 article from Consumer Reports. The ADA also promoted its message in a two-minute video news release sent to 700 TV stations on December 17, 1990, on its weekly radio show on December 18, 1990, and in its journal, the Journal of the American Dental Association.[174]

The same disgruntled reaction has repeated itself in more recent years. In January 2013, *The Doctors*, a national television show about topics of medical interest to the American public, aired an episode entitled "Dangerous Toxins."[175] The program highlighted the recovery of Stacy Case, a news anchor in

Nashville, TN, from multiple sclerosis after the safe removal of her dental amalgam fillings by an IAOMT member dentist.

The episode also featured a demonstration of the mercury vapors released from an amalgam filling by Dr. Boyd Haley. During the episode, Dr. Hewlett, an ADA spokesperson, attempted to invalidate Dr. Haley's work by announcing, "The types of data that he's reporting to you have not been replicated in peer-reviewed scientific studies."[176]

Research confirms [177] [178] [179] Dr. Haley's work, but Dr. Hewlett of the ADA apparently did not know that or did not want to admit it.

At any extent, another popular television show that aired a few months after *The Doctors* episode caused even more problems for the ADA. On a March 2013 segment of *The Dr. Oz Show* entitled "Are Your Silver Fillings Making Your Sick?," Dr. Oz, dentists, and other guests warned viewers of the potential dangers of dental mercury. [180]

The same day, the ADA issued a press release accusing Dr. Oz of "sensationalism" and declaring that "not one credible scientific study" shows dental mercury is a health risk. [181]

Yet again, the ADA failed to recognize hundreds of scientific studies. The ADA also failed to recognize that warnings on television programs might have become necessary since some would claim that the ADA has not protected consumers from dental amalgam.

WHAT ALTERNATIVES EXIST FOR TOOTH RESTORATIONS OTHER THAN DENTAL AMALGAM FILLINGS?

Considering all of the research about the harms of dental amalgam, one might be wondering what other choices exist for filling materials. There are several options available including gold alloys, indirect composites, glass ionomers, and ceramic (porcelain) dental materials, among other alternatives to amalgam.[182] Mercury-free restorations are described here:

Gold

Gold has been used in dentistry longer than amalgam and has been shown to be relatively biocompatible. However, the gold normally used in dentistry is an alloy. This means that it has been mixed with some other metal element such as palladium, copper, or cobalt, to give it certain structural characteristics. Thus, the actual percentage of gold contained in these alloys will vary from 2% to 92%, depending on the manufacturer and the price range desired.

As noted earlier in this booklet, mixing metals in the mouth can also contribute to health problems via oral galvinism, especially if gold fillings or crowns are placed near mercury amalgam fillings. Moreover, cheaper gold alloys often have base metals added, and these other metals can pose additional problems.[183]

Another main problem with gold is that it is expensive, and the price of dental gold normally fluctuates with the price of gold on the world market.

Composites (plastic resin fillings)

Whereas dental amalgam fillings have been called "silver" fillings because of their gray appearance, composite fillings are often called "white" fillings because of their tooth-like color. The appeal of having restorations that look natural has helped make composites one of the most popular fillings available today.

Composite materials are made of microscopic glass particles bound together by plastic resin. Originally used only for front teeth, they have been developed over the last 25 years into a class of products that is very suitable for use in back teeth. Compositions vary, but they all contain a variety of glass formulas and a variety of complex acrylic and urethane resins.

The newer composites being used for posterior restorations have been subjected to hundreds of research experiments to determine whether they are biocompatible and safe to use in the human body. Data produced by these studies indicates a very high degree of biocompatibility when properly placed.[184] [185]

Yet, because most of these composite fillings contain a form of bisphenol-A (BPA), a chemical that has been banned in some food containers and children's products, composite fillings have also been subject to scrutiny. Risk assessment scientist G. Mark Richardson, PhD, has extensively researched the biocompatibility of dental composites.[186][187] His work shows that patients with eight composites are exposed to levels of bisphenol-A that are 129 times LOWER than the exposure considered to be dangerous for estrogenic effects,[188] whereas patients with seven amalgam surfaces are exposed to quantities of mercury that are HIGHER than levels considered to be safe.[189]

Another aspect of composite fillings that has been criticized is their durability. However, several recent studies have notably debunked the claim that composites are not as durable as amalgam.[190][191][192]

Finally, a small percentage of people experience varying degrees of post-operative pain and thermal sensitivity (hot or cold) from composite fillings. A very common reason for this sensitivity is that the new filling is too high for the bite, especially for the molar teeth in the very back of the mouth. Having one's mouth opened widely for the filling replacement procedure sometimes causes a minor, temporary misalignment of the jaw which quickly returns to normal a few hours after the procedure. However, when the dentist is shaping the filling to conform to the bite, this temporary misalignment can mislead the dentist into thinking that the bite is good when it really is not. Most of the time, sensitivity that has not gone away after a couple of weeks can be eliminated simply by returning to the dentist for a quick adjustment of the bite.

Glass Ionomer

Another option that some dentists are using instead of amalgam fillings is temporary or interim fillings. In some situations, whether for personal health or financial reasons, glass ionomer fillings are put in place until they can be replaced with more permanent materials.

The option of glass ionomer is especially important when considering dental care in third-world or developing countries where access to dental tools is limited. This is because the Atraumatic Restorative Treatment (ART) technique for dental work requires only hand instruments and an adhesive restorative material such as glass ionomer cement for the dentist.[193] ART has been used successfully for decades in 25 countries and is even recommended by the World Health Organization.[194] [195]

Yet, controversy over glass ionomer fillings exists as well because glass ionomer fillings usually contain fluoride, which is another chemical that has been associated with toxic risks.

Ceramic (porcelain)

The use of ceramics as a restorative material for teeth is a rapidly growing option.

Whereas in the past ceramic fillings had to be shipped out and made in a laboratory, now new technology exists that allows dentists to construct the material at their office during a single patient appointment.

Ceramics have not been associated with any toxic side effects, but they can be more expensive than other alternatives in a price range with inlays and crowns. Fillings made by the older porcelain technology have been known in some cases to be more likely to facture than other materials, but the current high-strength ceramics are much more durable.

In conclusion, the potential for reaction exists with any foreign material implanted into the human body. To delineate what dental materials might work best for an individual, some dentists advocate using sensitivity or biocompatibility testing. Although these tests have yet to receive widespread support in the dental and medical professions, they are certainly worthy of consideration for patients with severe illnesses or compromised immune systems.

Although the final jury might still be out on what the best material for tooth restorations is, all present indications for mercury-free dentistry are promising. In fact, more than half of all dentists use resin composites or compomers instead of amalgam.[196] In this regard, there are several aspects of the newer restorative materials that are very encouraging:

(1) They do not contain mercury.

(2) They are esthetically pleasing. When a person smiles, others do not see black, gray, or silver areas. Instead, what is seen looks like the natural tooth color.

(3) The new materials are not known to generate any electrical currents and therefore do not appear to corrode any other metallic fillings or restorations in the mouth.

(4) There is less loss of natural tooth structure because the dentist does not have to do extensive preparation for the newer materials.

(5) The end result of using these newer materials is that they can truly be called restorations rather than fillings. This is because amalgam does not restore the tooth and can cause damage.

Unfortunately, and for far too long, dentistry has had to rely on potentially toxic materials for tooth restorations because there were no acceptable alternatives available. Now, modern technology and scientific advancements are providing a variety of materials, offering dental consumers the opportunity to evaluate what substances are implanted into their mouths.

WILL REPLACING DENTAL AMALGAM FILLINGS WITH ALTERNATIVE MATERIALS IMPROVE HEALTH?

While each patient's response varies, evidence supports the potential for a decrease of a variety of symptoms when dental amalgam fillings are **safely** removed. [197 198 199 200 201 202 203 204 205 206]

For example, statistics compiled by the Foundation for Toxic-Free Dentistry (FTFD) on 1569 patients from six different reports found improvements in a variety of health symptoms after the elimination of dental amalgam fillings, as the following table shows:

SELECTED HEALTH SYMPTOM ANALYSIS OF 1569 PATIENTS BEFORE AND AFTER ELIMINATION OF MERCURY FILLINGS

# of total patients report	% of total patients report	SYMPTOM or ISSUE	# of patients cured/ improved	% of patients cured/ improved
221	14	ALLERGY	196	89
86	5	ANXIETY	80	93
81	5	BAD TEMPER	68	89
88	6	BLOATING	70	88
99	6	BLOOD PRESSURE	53	54
79	5	CHEST PAINS	69	87
270	17	CONCENTRATION	216	80
347	22	DEPRESSION	315	91
343	22	DIZZINESS	301	88
705	45	FATIGUE	603	86
231	15	GASTROINTESTINAL	192	83
129	8	GUM PROBLEMS	121	94

# of total patients report	% of total patients report	SYMPTOM or ISSUE	# of patients cured/ improved	% of patients cured/ improved
531	34	HEADACHES	460	87
187	12	INSOMNIA	146	78
159	10	IRREG. HEARTBEAT	139	87
132	8	IRRITABILIY	119	90
91	6	LACK OF ENERGY	88	97
265	17	MEMORY LOSS	193	73
260	17	METALLIC TASTE	247	95
45	3	MIGRAINES	39	87
113	7	MULTIPLE SCLEROSIS	86	76
126	8	MUSCLE TREMOR	104	83
158	10	NERVOUSNESS	131	83
118	8	NUMBNESS	97	82
310	20	SKIN DISTURBANCE	251	81
149	9	SORE THROAT	128	86
97	6	TACHYCARDIA	68	70
56	4	THYROID	44	79
189	12	ULCERS/SORES (ORAL)	162	86
115	7	URINARY TRACT	87	76
462	29	VISION	289	63

Considering the wide-range of symptoms related to mercury, it is interesting that a report entitled *The Economics of Dental Amalgam Regulation* noted: "We can then make the case that the overall health care expenditures necessary to deal with diseases and conditions, known or unknown, arising from the continued installation of amalgam could far exceed the relatively manageable cost increases to the consumer for the alternatives…This is not to mention the cost to the U.S. economy of lost work time owing to concomitant illness and disability." [207]

IS REPLACING DENTAL AMALGAM FILLNGS DANGEROUS?

There is a risk of additional mercury exposure to dentists, dental staff, and patients from any and all unsafe procedures involving mercury amalgam fillings, especially if treatment, hygiene routines, removal, and/or replacement of fillings are conducted without taking appropriate protective measures. However, if safe practices are applied, mercury exposure can be drastically decreased in all of these scenarios.

This concept is essential to understand because as long as dental amalgam is used in dentistry and is still in the mouths of patients, maintenance and removal of dental amalgam will be necessary, especially because amalgam fillings wear out over time. Data has shown that "amalgam restorations have a 50% failure time between 5.5 to 11.5 years,"[208] and in six-year-old children, the median survival time for occlusal amalgam fillings in first permanent molars is twenty-six months.[209]

Most fillings are replaced because of decay under the filling, excessive corrosion, fracture, etc. The procedure is so commonplace that many insurance companies will pay for replacement of an amalgam filling after only one year.

Safety measures during the amalgam removal procedure

When it comes to the removal of amalgam fillings, there are special techniques that can be utilized by the dentist to make the procedure safer. If these techniques are applied properly, there is less exposure to the increased levels of mercury vapor caused by the removal procedure.

Therefore, it is important for patients to be aware of certain aspects related to safe amalgam removal:
1. The dentist should have an assistant present to assist in minimizing exposure to any mercury vapor, thus protecting both the dental staff and the patient. The correct protocol requires the use of large volumes of cold water both from the drill and from separate irrigation by the assistant, who should also be simultaneously using high volume suction evacuation on the

vapor and particles released during the removal procedure. The assistant should hold the high volume evacuator positioned next to the tooth being worked on until all of the cut filling and cavity have been cleaned out.

2. Mercury vapor pressure doubles with every ten degree Centigrade rise in temperature, which is extremely important considering the friction from drilling generates significant temperature increases. One procedure that minimizes extensive drilling involves sectioning the amalgam into chunks versus just drilling the entire filling out all at once.

3. In some dental offices, the dentist may ask the patient to breathe through a nose piece that permits the patient to draw air from another area so as not to inhale mercury vapor released during the removal process. Sometimes, oxygen masks are also used over the nose for breathing.

4. During amalgam removal, the dentist and assistant are at a high risk from exposure to mercury spray and vapor. They should be wearing special clothing, masks, and surgical gloves, which should be handled properly after the procedure is completed. These measures protect them from excessive exposure to mercury during repeated removal operations and protect areas where mercury could be transported to via contaminated clothing, etc.

5. Some dentists will have the patient wear a rubber dam during the amalgam removal procedure. This is a square of rubber stretched on a frame that isolates the tooth or teeth being

worked on. The rubber dam is supposed to prevent the patient from swallowing drilled out amalgam particles and/or accidentally inhaling mercury fumes. However, high levels of mercury vapor have been measured under rubber dams, and if a dentist uses a rubber dam, the patient should be sure to breathe through the nose instead of the mouth during the removal process. Additionally, some dentists specify using a non-latex dam because they are less permeable to mercury vapor.

6. The office should be well-ventilated, which is why many mercury-free dentists are now installing central vacuuming systems in their offices. Patients might be asked to hold the vacuum hose on their chests during the removal process. Some doctors have even added "Air Purifying Systems" to eliminate or reduce these background levels of mercury in the office.

Regardless of the precautions outlined, some individuals may experience reactions to mercury released during the removal procedures. These are described as being flu-like and can last from one to seven days. Symptoms can include fever, nausea, headaches, etc. If such symptoms persist, patients should be sure to let their dentist and trusted health care professional know.

Dietary and nutritional safety measures

Nutritional measures, diet modification, and the addition of certain supplements are often recommended to reduce the toxic effects of mercury from sources other than dental amalgam and to assist the individual's body in coping with any mercury exposure from the removal procedure.

Diet modification usually involves attempting to reduce the amount of mercury ingested such as fish and other foods with high mercury content. Reduction of refined carbohydrates and sugars is also beneficial, as harmful oral and gut bacteria seem to thrive on these types of food. Furthermore, increasing dietary fiber intake helps by inducing a faster transit time of waste matter and toxins to be excreted. The same is true of increasing water intake to assist the body in flushing out toxins through the kidneys.

Nutritional supplements should be suggested only if scientific research has shown that they can help the body excrete mercury by binding with it and/or by neutralizing some of the biochemical byproducts created when mercury impacts normal metabolic processes.

Chelation

There are also therapeutic chelating protocols available. Chelating products are designed to help detoxify the human system by binding to mercury and other heavy metals and assisting in their release from the body. Chelation is a very complex process, and new research related to chelation is continually developing.

There are a number of products and supplements often used in chelation including DMSA, DMPS, EDTA, Vitamin C, chlorella, cilantro, and alpha lipoic acid. Additionally, some detoxifiers are specifically designed to raise levels of glutathione and/or relieve oxidative stress.

Chelating options should be researched thoroughly, and chelation should only be used by a patient under the care of a qualified physician because adverse reactions to chelating agents are possible.

Sweat therapy

The medical text book "Environmental and Occupational Medicine"[210] indicates that sweat induction may also be of therapeutic value in reducing the total body burden of mercury. Historically, Spanish groups used sweat therapy on workers in mercury mines who exhibited signs or symptoms of mercury vapor toxicity.[211]

Any means of inducing sweating appears to be acceptable, including steam baths, saunas, heat lamps, exercise, etc. Using sweat therapy is supposed to increase the elimination of mercury through the skin and should therefore help in reducing the total body burden.

As with other forms of chelation, all patients, especially pregnant women or anyone with a history of cardiovascular problems, should obtain assistance from their physician prior to undertaking routine sweat therapy.

Overall, it is essential for individuals to discuss amalgam removal techniques and safety measures with their dentists and with their physicians (especially in the event a physician has suggested amalgam removal because of suspected mercury toxicity).

HOW CAN I FIND OUT IF THE MERCURY COMING OUT OF MY DENTAL AMALGAM FILLINGS IS HURTING ME OR IF I AM HYPERSENSITIVE TO IT?

Mercury exposure and mercury burden testing

Obviously, in the case of dental amalgam, it is difficult to measure or detect mercury that has been stored in tissues and organs over time. Thus, this is a complex area that is developing with modern science. While there is no overall consensus on the best way to accurately calculate levels of mercury within the human body and where that mercury is being stored, new tests are offering advanced methods to make this possible.

For years, the ADA maintained that urine and blood tests for mercury content were a valid means of determining safe exposure levels and dangerous exposure levels. However, after the 1984 Workshop on the Biocompatibility of

Metals in Dentistry, the ADA finally agreed with the overwhelming scientific evidence (existent since the early 1960's) indicating that blood and urine tests are invalid for determining toxicity or cellular damage that may be occurring in the body.

Typical blood and urine tests can, however, indicate whether an exposure to mercury occurred, and generally speaking, these tests are most useful immediately after a major exposure to mercury, such as an industrial accident.

Mercury allergy and sensitivity testing

It is easily possible to be tested for mercury allergies and sensitivities. One of the traditional methods utilized by the medical profession to determine hypersensitivity is the use of skin patch testing. Dilute concentrations of the suspected allergen are applied to the skin by the use of a patch or injection. There is considerable controversy concerning this procedure because the patch test can greatly exacerbate a patient's symptoms if the individual is allergic or highly sensitive to mercury.

Yet, modern science is changing the course of these tests as well, and past practices are being replaced with innovative new tests. One alternative to skin patch testing for metal sensitivity is known as the Lymphocyte Transformation Test (LTT).[212] This blood test is gaining popularity because it does not expose patients to the same materials that could be making them ill.

Patient medical history

The single most important diagnostic tool is the patient. It is integral for dentists to listen to the patient, especially about symptoms that could be related to mercury and/or their dental fillings. It is likewise important that the patient feels comfortable discussing health concerns with the dentist. If the dentist does not know about an issue, nothing can be done to address it.

HOW EXPENSIVE ARE THE ALTERNATIVE MATERIALS AND WILL INSURANCE PLANS PAY FOR THEM?

At the present time, the price the dentist pays for non-mercury materials is more than the price of the amalgam. Coupled with this higher material cost is the necessity to use a technique-sensitive procedure that requires the dentist to spend more time with the patient to properly place and bond the material to the tooth. The net result is a higher unit cost per surface for composite restorations versus amalgam fillings.

What this means is that some insurance companies refuse to pay for composite fillings because they will only pay the comparable cost of an amalgam filling. The patient then has to pay the difference in cost between the amalgam filling and the composite filling.

Many believe that the basis for non-payment is largely due to the fact that the ADA has been critical of the use of composites in posterior teeth,[213] a move that has kept many dentists using amalgam in those areas of the mouth. It would appear that the ADA has an agenda for non-approval of composites that embraces reasons other than product quality and acceptability. It is probably not just a coincidence that dental establishments in several countries have maintained that they will replace the use of amalgam when suitable posterior composites are available.

Concerns about the failure of insurance carriers to pay for mercury-free alternatives have recently been expressed in a legal journal. A 2013 article in the *Boston College Journal of Law & Social Justice* by Kaitlin McGrath states:

> Additionally, because Medicaid does not cover alternative fillings, many low-income Americans are forced to choose between mercury fillings or no fillings at all. Although other countries have banned or severely restricted the use of mercury fillings, the United States has yet to enact federal legislation on the issue. This Note argues that Congress should

ban mercury fillings or, at a minimum, implement uniform warning requirements and mandate insurance and Medicaid coverage for alternative fillings.[214]

The need for insurance reform to include mercury-free alternatives in coverage has even been addressed by the United Nations Environment Programme's Mimamata Convention on Mercury. The international mercury treaty, signed by over 90 counties (including the United States) in 2013, calls for "discouraging insurance policies and programmes that favour dental amalgam use over mercury-free dental restoration" and "encouraging insurance policies and programmes that favour the use of quality alternatives to dental amalgam for dental restoration."[215]

If an insurance company will not pay full price for composite restorations, the patient should register a written complaint with the State Insurance Commissioner, his or her employer, and the insurance company. Employers are urged to shop around for a carrier who will provide full coverage for biocompatible non-metal restorative materials and who will support the constitutional right to freedom of choice. If a payment on a pre-submittal claim related to amalgam replacement for health reasons is refused, an attorney should write a letter to the insurance carrier requesting that they have their corporate attorney respond in writing. The corporate attorney's response should state that the insurance carrier assumes all liability for health problems that may result from the continued release of mercury vapor from the dental amalgam in the patient's mouth.

WHAT IS INFORMED CONSENT?

According to the American Medical Association (AMA), informed consent is "a process of communication between a patient and physician that results in the patient's authorization or agreement to undergo a specific medical intervention."[216] The AMA also establishes that informed consent should involve a discussion about risks, benefits, and alternatives, regardless of what is covered in the individual's health care plan.

Informed consent requirements for procedures involving dental restorations have been passed in California,[217] Connecticut,[218] Maine,[219] and Vermont,[220] and each of these states has some type of brochure that dental patients are supposed to receive which explains their options for tooth restorations and risks associated with mercury.

Included in Appendix A of this book is a sample of an Informed Consent form. It has been designed to be used in conjunction with this book.

IN CONCLUSION…

The intent of the explanations offered in this booklet is to insure that the patient has sufficient information to make a decision as to which materials are placed in his or her teeth and/or the teeth of his or her children. Patients should also understand no claims can be made that removal and replacement of mercury amalgam fillings will cure any known disease or eliminate or modify any symptoms. Additionally, while scientific studies suggest that dental amalgam is a potential factor in causing or exacerbating a variety of health conditions, there are no studies conclusively identifying dental amalgam mercury as the main culprit in these illnesses.

Although we are routinely subjected to mercury intake from the environment and our food chain, these are sources essentially beyond our personal control. However, opting for mercury-free fillings is within our individual jurisdiction, and it reduces the mercury exposure taken on by an individual. The less mercury is used in dentistry, the less it is used in the world, which creates a healthier future for patients and dental workers, their children, and the world at large.

APPENDIX A: INFORMED CONSENT FORM

I, _____, give

my dentist,_____ permission

to remove serviceable dental amalgam fillings and other non-precious metals from my teeth and replace them with dental materials considered to be biocompatible based on existing scientific research. These materials may include, but are not limited to, composite resins, ceramic, porcelain, gold alloys, glass ionomers, and titanium.

My dentist has provided me with a personal copy of the booklet *Dentistry without Mercury*, which explains the pros and cons on the use of amalgam as a dental material and also gives the position of the American Dental Association on the safety of dental amalgam. Any questions I had that were not answered by this booklet were subsequently answered to my satisfaction by my dentist.

My dentist has explained to me that: 1) Although one or more of my subjective or objective signs or symptoms may resemble the signs or symptoms of mercury toxicity, this does not mean that I am suffering from the effects of mercury toxicity either directly or indirectly. 2) There is no specific, conclusive scientific evidence that removal of my amalgam dental fillings will positively cure or improve any signs, symptoms, problems, or health conditions that I have. 3) Any sign, symptom, problem, or health condition that I have outside the mouth might involve a general health or medical question. My dentist is limiting advice to the mouth and recommends that I consult a physician for any general health or medical concerns or questions which I have.

4) Further, my dentist has not told me or represented to me that replacing my amalgam fillings or non-precious metals would have any beneficial health effect on me at all. If a posterior composite resin is the material chosen to replace dental amalgam and other non-precious materials,

the advantages and disadvantages of the material chosen have been explained to me.

As might occur with the placement of amalgam, gold, or any other dental material, I understand that there are situations beyond the control of my dentist that could necessitate endodontic treatment or removal of an existing tooth despite precautions taken and proper procedures utilized. In addition, I understand that during the removal and replacement of dental materials, an allergic type reaction to products used that could require immediate treatment is possible. There is also a more delayed allergic reaction which is like a general sickness. Should I begin feeling poorly, I understand that it is my responsibility to advise my dentist immediately and to seek medical treatment.

My questions concerning the treatment plan recommended by my dentist and agreed to by me have been fully answered, and I have read this statement and am satisfied that I have been fully informed.

Patient
Signature:_____

Patient
Printed Name: _____

Dentist
Name: _____

Witness
Signature: _____

Witness
Printed Name:_____

Date: _____

APPENDIX B:
MORE INFORMATION ABOUT
THE INTERNATIONAL ACADEMY OF
ORAL MEDICINE AND TOXICOLOGY
(IAOMT)

Founded in 1984, the International Academy of Oral Medicine and Toxicology (IAOMT) is a worldwide organization of dentists, physicians, and research professionals devoted to the examination, compilation, and dissemination of scientific information about the biocompatibility of oral/dental materials. The fundamental mission of the IAOMT is to promote the health of the public. In this regard, the IAOMT continually reviews, composes, and shares analytical research and educational materials related to the biocompatibility of oral/dental materials.

Information about finding an IAOMT dentist in your area and access to more details about the IAOMT's mission and documents applicable to this booklet are available from the IAOMT.

Contact information for IAOMT:
8297 ChampionsGate Blvd, #193
ChampionsGate, FL 33896
Email: info@iaomt.org
Telephone: (863) 420-6373
Fax: (863) 419-8136

Website: www.iaomt.org

APPENDIX C:
MORE INFORMATION ABOUT
DENTAL AMALGAM
MERCURY SOLUTIONS, INC. (DAMS)

Some concerned citizens, most of them prior victims of mercury poisoning from their dental amalgam fillings, have formed victim support groups around the country. The dedicated individuals involved in DAMS are largely volunteers who aim to provide understanding and information to those individuals bewildered by their health conditions and those who are trying to gain additional knowledge about the potential health effects of mercury. DAMS also works to protect the right of mercury-free dentists to continue practicing. The staff at the main DAMS office can help patients find qualified holistic dentists in their state or province. Upon request, DAMS will send interested individuals an information packet that includes a current Dental Health Guide, a list of DAMS professional members and, if available, additional resources.

Contact information for DAMS:
DAMS
1043 Grand Ave, #317
St Paul, MN 55105
Email: dams@usfamily.net
Telephone: (651) 644-4572

ENDNOTES

[1] World Health Organization. Mercury in Health Care [policy paper]. Geneva, Switzerland: WHO; August 2005.
http://www.who.int/water_sanitation_health/medicalwaste/mercurypolpaper.pdf.

[2] Health Canada. *The Safety of Dental Amalgam.* Ottawa, Ontario: Minister of Health; 1996.

[3] Reuters/PRNewswire-USNewswire Online. Dental mercury use banned in Norway, Sweden and Denmark because composites are adequate replacements [press release]. January 3, 2008.
http://www.reuters.com/article/idUS108558+03-Jan-2008+PRN20080103.

[4] Orthomolecular Medicine News Service. Mercury dental amalgams banned in 3 countries: FDA, EPA, ADA still allow and encourage heavy-metal fillings [press release]. November 20, 2008.
http://orthomolecular.org/resources/omns/v04n24.shtml.

[5] Health and Environment Alliance. Mercury and Dental Amalgams [fact sheet]. Brussels, Belgium: Health and Environment Alliance and Health Care without Harm; May 2007: 3. http://www.env-health.org/IMG/pdf/HEA_009-07.pdf.

[6] Health and Environment Alliance. Mercury and Dental Amalgams [fact sheet] Brussels, Belgium; Health and Environment Alliance and Health Care without Harm; May 2007: 3. http://www.env-health.org/IMG/pdf/HEA_009-07.pdf.

[7] United Nations Environment Programme. Minamata Convention on Mercury. Geneva, Switzerland: Text agreed upon in UNEP(DTIE)/Hg/INC.5/3; January 13-19, 2013.
http://www.mercuryconvention.org/Portals/11/documents/conventionText/Minamata%20Convention%20on%20Mercury_e.pdf

[8] Dental Board of California. The Facts about Fillings [fact sheet]. Sacramento, CA: California Department of Consumer Affairs; 5/04.

http://www.dbc.ca.gov/formspubs/pub_dmfs_english_we
bview.pdf.

[9] State of Connecticut Department of Environmental
Protection. Fillings: The Choices You Have: Mercury
Amalgam and Other Filling Materials [brochure].
Hartford, CT: DEP; May 2011.
http://www.ct.gov/dep/lib/dep/mercury/gen_info/fillings_
brochure.pdf.

[10] Maine Bureau of Health. Filling Materials [brochure].
Augusta, ME: Bureau of Health, 2002.
http://www.vce.org/mercury/Maine_AmalBrochFinal2.pd
f

[11] Advisory Committee on Mercury Pollution. Dental
Amalgam Fillings: Environmental and Health Facts for
Dental Patients [brochure]. Waterbury, Vermont:
Mercury Education and Reduction Campaign.
http://www.mercvt.org/PDF/DentalAmalgamFactSheet.pd
f. Accessed August 22, 2013.

[12] Richardson GM, Wilson R, Allard D, Purtill C, Douma
S, Gravière, J. Mercury exposure and risks from dental
amalgam in the US population, post-2000. *Science of the
Total Environment.* 2011; 409(20):4257-4268.

[13] Hahn LJ, Kloiber R, Vimy MJ, Takahashi Y,
Lorscheider F. Dental "silver" tooth fillings: a source of
mercury exposure revealed by whole-body image scan
and tissue analysis. *FASEB J.* 1989; 3(14):2641-2646.

[14] Vimy MJ, Lorscheider FL. Serial measurements of
intra-oral air mercury: estimation of daily dose from
dental amalgam. *J Dent Res.* 1985; 64(8):1072-5.

[15] Vimy MJ, Lorscheider FL. Clinical science intra-oral
air mercury released from dental amalgam. *J Den Res.*
1985; 64(8):1069-71.

[16] Weiner JA, Nylander M, Berglund F. Does mercury
from amalgam restorations constitute a health hazard? *Sci
Total Environ.* 1990: 99(1-2):1-22.

[17] Richardson GM, Brecher RW, Scobie H, Hamblen J,
Samuelian J, Smith C. Mercury vapour (Hg(0)):
Continuing toxicological uncertainties, and establishing a

Canadian reference exposure level. *Regul Toxicol Pharmicol.* February 2009; 53(1):32-38.

[18] Richardson GM. Inhalation of mercury-contaminated particulate matter by dentists: an overlooked occupational risk. *Human and Ecological Risk Assessment.* 2003; 9(6):1519-1531.

[19] Snapp KR, Svare CW, Peterson LD. Contribution of dental amalgams to blood mercury levels. *J Dent Res.* 1981; 65(special issue):311, Abstract #1276.

[20] Nimmo A, Werley MS, Martin JS, Tansy MF. Particulate inhalation during the removal of amalgam restorations. *J Prosth Dent.* 1990; 63(2):228-33.

[21] Reinhardt JW. Side-effects: Mercury contribution to body burden from dental amalgam. *Adv Dent Res.* 1992; 6(1):110-3.

[22] Stonehouse CA, Newman AP. Mercury vapour release from a dental aspirator. *Br Dent J.* 2001; 190(10):558-560.

[23] Gay DD, Cox RD, Reinhardt JW: Chewing releases mercury from fillings. *Lancet.* 1979; 313(8123):985-6.

[24] Krausß, P., M. Deyhle, K. H. Maier, E. Roller, H. D. Weiß, and Ph Clédon. Field study on the mercury content of saliva. *Toxicological & Environmental Chemistry.* 1997; 63, (1-4):29-46.

[25] Isacsson G, Barregard L, Selden A, Bodin L. Impact of nocturnal bruxism on mercury uptake from dental amalgams. *Eur J Oral Sci.* 1997; 105(3):251-7.

[26] Sallsten G, Thoren J, Barregard L, Schutz A, Skarping G. Long-term use of nicotine chewing gum and mercury exposure from dental amalgam fillings. *J Dent Res.* 1996; 75(1):594-8.

[27] Björkman L, Lind B. Factors influencing mercury evaporation rate from dental amalgam fillings. *Scand J Dent Res.* 1992; 100(6):354-60.

[28] Richardson GM. Inhalation of mercury-contaminated particulate matter by dentists: an overlooked occupational risk. *Human and Ecological Risk Assessment.* 2003; 9(6): 1519-1531.

[29] Health Canada. *The Safety of Dental Amalgam.* Ottawa, Ontario: Minister of Health; 1996.

[30] Sandborgh-Englund G, Elinder CG, Langworth S, Schutz A, Ekstrand J. Mercury in biological fluids after amalgam removal. *J Dent Res.* 1998; 77(4):615-24.

[31] Nimmo A, Werley MS, Martin JS, Tansy MF. Particulate inhalation during the removal of amalgam restorations. *J Prosth Dent.* 1990; 63(2):228-33.

[32] Skare I. Mercury exposure from amalgam: a background study *National Board of Occupational Safety and Health. S-17184 Solna, Sweden. Abstr Scand Occup Hygiene Meet. Iceland.* 1987.

[33] Richardson GM, Wilson R, Allard D, Purtill C, Douma S, Gravière J. Mercury exposure and risks from dental amalgam in the US population, post-2000. *Science of the Total Environment.* 2011; 409(20):4257-4268.

[34] Reinhardt JW. Side-effects: Mercury contribution to body burden from dental amalgam. *Adv Dent Res.* 1992; 6(1):110-3.

[35] Björkman L, Sandborgh-Englund G, Ekstrand J. Mercury in saliva and feces after removal of amalgam fillings. *Toxicol Appl Pharmacol.* 1997; 144(1):156–62.

[36] Stock A, Cucuel F. Der Quecksilbergehalt der menschlichen Ausscheidungen und des menschlichen Blutes. *Angewandte Chemie.* 1934; 47(37):641-647.

[37] Frykholm KO. *On Mercury from Dental Amalgam: Its Toxic and Allergic Effects, and Some Comments on Occupational Hygiene.* Almqvist & Wiksells boktr.; 1957.

[38] Stortebecker P. *Mercury Poisoning from Dental Amalgam -a Hazard to Human Brain.* Orlando, FL: Bio-Probe, Inc.; 1985:32-43.

[39] Mercury: Human Exposure. United States Environmental Protection Agency Web site. http://www.epa.gov/hg/exposure.htm. Updated July 9, 2013.

[40] United States Food and Drug Administration, United States Environmental Protection Agency. What You Need to Know about Mercury in Fish and Shellfish

[brochure EPA-823-R-04-005]. Washington, D.C.: FDA and EPA; March 2004. http://www.fda.gov/Food/ResourcesForYou/Consumers/ucm110591.htm.

[41] Sellars WA, Sllars R, Liang L, Hefley JD. Methyl mercury in dental amalgams in the human mouth. *Journal of Nutritional and Environmental Medicine*. 1996; 6(1):33-36.

[42] Heintze U, Edwardsson S, Derand T, Birkhed D. Methylation of mercury from dental amalgam and mercuric chloride by oral streptococci in vitro. *European Journal of Oral Sciences*. 1983; 91(2):150-152.

[43] Wang J, Liu Z. In vitro study of streptococcus mutans in the plaque on the surface of amalgam fillings on the conversion of inorganic mercury to organic mercury. *Shanghai Kou Qiang Yi Xue*. 2002; 9(2):70-72.

[44] Leistevuo J, Leistevuo T, Helenius H, Pyy L, Österblad M, Huovinen P, Tenovuo. Dental amalgam fillings and the amount of organic mercury in human saliva. *Caries Research*. 2001; 35(3):163-166.

[45] Rowland IR, Grasso P, Davies MJ. The methylation of mercuric chloride by human intestinal bacteria. *Cellular and Molecular Life Sciences*. 1975; 31(9):1064-5.

[46] Yannai S, Berdicevsky I, Duek L. Transformations of inorganic mercury by candida albicans and saccharomyces cerevisiae. *Applied and Environmental Microbiology*. 1991; 57(1):245-247.

[47] Summers AO, Wireman J, Vimy MJ, Lorscheider FL, Marshall B, Levy SB, Billard L. Mercury released from dental "silver" fillings provokes an increase in mercury- and antibiotic-resistant bacteria in oral and intestinal floras of primates. *Antimicrobial agents and chemotherapy*. 1993; 37(4):825-834.

[48] Schriever W, Diamond LE. Electromotive forces and electric currents caused by metallic dental fillings. *J Dent Res*. 1952. 31(2):205-228.

[49] Schneider PE, Sarker NK. Mercury release from dispersalloy amalgam. *IADR Abstract #630*. 1982.

[50] Phillips R.W. *Skinner's Science of Dental Materials* (7th ed). Philadelphia, PA: W.B. Saunders Co., 1973.
[51] Pigatto PDM, Brambilla L, Ferrucci S, Guzzi G. Systemic Allergic Contact dermatitis due to galvanic couple between mercury amalgam and titanium implant. *Skin Allergy Meeting*. 2010.
[52] Hyams BL, Ballon HC. Dissimilar metals in the mouth as a possible cause of otherwise unexplainable symptoms. *Canadian Medical Association Journal*. 1933; 29(5):488.
[53] Richardson GM, Brecher RW, Scobie H, Hamblen J, Samuelian J, Smith C. Mercury vapour (Hg(0)): Continuing toxicological uncertainties, and establishing a Canadian reference exposure level. *Regul Toxicol Pharmicol*. 2009; 53(1):32-38.
[54] Mutter J, Naumann J, Walach H, Daschner F. Amalgam risk assessment with coverage of references up to 2005. *Gesundheitswesen*. 2005; 67(3):204-216.
[55] Advisory Committee on Mercury Pollution. Dental Amalgam Fillings: Environmental and Health Facts for Dental Patients [brochure]. Waterbury, Vermont: Mercury Education and Reduction Campaign. http://www.mercvt.org/PDF/DentalAmalgamFactSheet.pdf. Accessed August 22, 2013.
[56] Maine Bureau of Health. Filling Materials [brochure]. Augusta, ME: Bureau of Health, 2002. http://www.vce.org/mercury/Maine_AmalBrochFinal2.pdf.
[57] State of Connecticut Department of Environmental Protection. Fillings: The Choices You Have: Mercury Amalgam and Other Filling Materials [brochure]. Hartford, CT: DEP; May 2011. http://www.ct.gov/dep/lib/dep/mercury/gen_info/fillings_brochure.pdf.
[58] Vimy MJ, Lorscheider FL. Clinical science intra-oral air mercury released from dental amalgam. *J Den Res*. 1985; 64(8):1069-71.
[59] Watson, Diane, and 18 other members of Congress. *Dear Acting Commissioner Dr. Joshua Sharfstein...* [Congressional letter]. Washington, D.C.: May 14, 2009.

Copy of letter available upon request to
john.donnelly@mail.house.gov.

[60] Watson, Diane (Congresswoman). *Mercury in Dental Filling Disclosure and Prohibition Act*. Los Angeles, CA: November 5, 2001. Copy of Act available at http://amalgamillness.com/Text_DCAct.html.

[61] Palkovicova L, Ursinyova M, Masanova V, Yu Z, Hertz-Picciotto I. Maternal amalgam dental fillings as the source of mercury exposure in developing fetus and newborn. *J Expo Sci Environ Epidemiol.* 2008; 18(3):326–31.

[62] Lutz E, Lind B, Herin P, Krakau I, Bui TH, Vahter M. Concentrations of mercury, cadmium and lead in brain and kidney of second trimester fetuses and infants. *J Trace Elem Med Biol.* 1996; 10(2):61–7.

[63] Geier DA, Kern JK, Geier MR. A prospective study of prenatal mercury exposure from dental amalgams and autism severity. *Neurobiolgiae Experimentals Polish Neuroscience Society.* 2009; 69(2):189-197.

[64] Ask K, Akesson A, Berglund M, Vahter M. Inorganic mercury and methylmercury in placentas of Swedish women. *Environ Health Perspect* 2002; 110(5):523-6.

[65] Vahter M, Akesson A, Lind B, Bjors U, Schutz A, Berglund M. Longitudinal study of methylmercury and inorganic mercury in blood and urine of pregnant and lactating women, as well as in umbilical cord blood. *Environ Res.* 2000; 84(2):186-94.

[66] da Costa SL, Malm O, Dórea JG. Breast-milk mercury concentrations and amalgam surface in mothers from Brasilia, Brazil. *Biol Trace Elem Res.* 2005; 106(2):145–51.

[67] Oskarsson A, Schutz A, Schkerving S, Hallen IP, Ohlin B, Lagerkvist BJ. Total and inorganic mercury in breast milk in relation to fish consumption and amalgam in lactating women. *Arch Environ Health.* 1996; 51(3):234-51.

[68] Nourouzi E, Bahramifar N, Ghasempouri SM. Effect of teeth amalgam on mercury levels in the colostrums

human milk in Lenjan. *Environ Monit Assess.* 2012; 184(1):375-380.

[69] Geier DA, Carmody T, Kern JK, King PG, Geier MR. A dose-dependent relationship between mercury exposure from dental amalgams and urinary mercury levels: a further assessment of the Casa Pia Children's Dental Amalgam Trial. *Human & experimental toxicology.* 2012; 31(1):11-17.

[70] Geier DA, Carmody T, Kern JK, King PG, Geier MR. A significant relationship between mercury exposure from dental amalgams and urinary porphyrins: a further assessment of the Casa Pia children's dental amalgam trial. *Biometals.* 2011; 24, (2):215-224.

[71] Woods JS, Heyer NJ, Echeverria D, Russo JE, Martin MD, Bernardo MF, Luis HS, Vaz L, Farin FM. Modification of neurobehavioral effects of mercury by a genetic polymorphism of coproporphyrinogen oxidase in children. *Neurotoxicol Teratol.* 2012; 34(5):513-21.

[72] Al-Saleh I, Al-Sedairi A. Mercury (Hg) burden in children: The impact of dental amalgam. *Sci Total Environ.* 2011; 409(16):3003-3015.

[73] Bellinger DC, Trachtenberg F; Barregard L, Tavares M, Cernichiari E, Daniel D, McKinlay S. Neuropyschological and renal effects of dental amalgam in children: a randomized clinical trial. *JAMA.* 2006; 295(15):1775-1783.

[74] DeRouen TA, Martin MD, Leroux BG, Townes BD, Woods JS, Leitão J, Castro-Caldas A, et al. Neurobehavioral effects of dental amalgam in children: a randomized clinical trial. *JAMA.* 2006; 295(15):1784-1792.

[75] Roberts, Allison. Portugal shamed by child sex case. *Sunday Herald.* October 12, 2003.

[76] Duffy S. Critique of the Children's Amalgam Study Consent Forms (American forms and Portuguese forms). IAOMT Web site. http://iaomt.guiadmin.com/wp-content/uploads/CAT_Duffy_legal_critique.pdf. Written June 16, 2004. Accessed August 25, 2013.

[77] Haley, BE. Response to the NIDCR Funded Children's Amalgam Testing publications in the JAMA 2006. IAOMT Web site. http://iaomt.guiadmin.com/wp-content/uploads/CAT_Haley_scientific_critique.pdf. Accessed August 25, 2013.

[78] Geier DA, Carmody T, Kern JK, King PG, Geier MR. A significant relationship between mercury exposure from dental amalgams and urinary porphyrins: a further assessment of the Casa Pia children's dental amalgam trial. *Biometals.* 2011; 24, (2):215-224.

[79] United States of America Department of Health and Human Services Food and Drug Administration, Center for Devices and Radiological Health Medical Devices Committee. Dental Products Panel [transcript]. December 15, 2010: 271. http://www.fda.gov/downloads/AdvisoryCommittees/CommitteesMeetingMaterials/MedicalDevices/MedicalDevicesAdvisoryCommittee/DentalProductsPanel/UCM242363.pdf

[80] Health and Environment Alliance. Mercury and Dental Amalgams [fact sheet]. Brussels, Belgium: Health and Environment Alliance and Health Care without Harm; May 2007: 3. http://www.env-health.org/IMG/pdf/HEA_009-07.pdf.

[81] Richardson GM. Inhalation of mercury-contaminated particulate matter by dentists: an overlooked occupational risk. *Human and Ecological Risk Assessment.* 2003; 9(6):1519-1531.

[82] Nimmo A, Werley MS, Martin JS, Tansy MF. Particulate inhalation during the removal of amalgam restorations. *J Prosth Dent.* 1990; 63(2):228-33.

[83] Sikorski R, Juszkiewicz T, Paszkowski T, Szprengier-Juszkiewicz T. Women in dental surgeries: reproductive hazards in exposure to metallic mercury. *International Archives of Occupational and Environmental Health.* 1987; 59(6):551-557.

[84] Rowland AS, Baird DD, Weinberg CR, Shore DL, Shy CM, Wilcox AJ. The effect of occupational exposure to

mercury vapour on the fertility of female dental assistants. *Occupat Environ Med.* 1994; 51:28-34.

[85] Buchwald H. Exposure of dental workers to mercury. *American Industrial Hygiene Association Journal.* 1972; 33(7):492-502.

[86] International Academy of Oral Medicine and Toxicology. Amalgam-Mercury Fact Sheet. IAOMT Web site: http://iaomt.guiadmin.com/wp-content/uploads/IAOMT-Fact-Sheet.pdf. Published August 5, 2011. Accessed August 25, 2013.

[87] Finne KAJ, Göransson K, Winckler L. Oral lichen planus and contact allergy to mercury. *International journal of oral surgery.* 1982; 11(4):236-239.

[88] Tomka M, Machovkova A, Pelclova D, Petanova J, Arenbergerova M, Prochazkova J. Orofacial granulomatosis associated with hypersensitivity to dental amalgam. *Science Direct.* 2011; 112(3):335-341.

[89] Lundstrom, IM. Allergy and corrosion of dental materials in patients with oral lichen planus. *Int J Oral Surg.* 1984; 13(1):16.

[90] Laine, J, Kalimo K, Forssell H, Happonen R. Resolution of oral lichenoid lesions after replacement of amalgam restorations in patients allergic to mercury compounds. *JAMA.* 1992; 267(21):2880.

[91] Lind PO, Hurlen B, Lyberg T, Aas E. Amalgam-related oral lichenoid reaction. *Scand J Dent Res.* 1986; 94(5):448-51.

[92] Pang BK, Freeman S. Oral lichenoid lesions caused by allergy to mercury in amalgam fillings. *Contact Dermatitis.* 1995; 33(6):423-7.

[93] White RR, Brandt RL. Development of mercury hypersensitivity among dental students. *JADA.* 1976; 92(6):1204-7.

[94] Godfrey ME, Wojcik DP, Krone CA. Apolipoprotein E genotyping as a potential biomarker for mercury toxicity. *Journal of Alzheimer's Disease.* 2003; 5(3): 189-195.

[95] Haley BE. Mercury toxicity: genetic susceptibility and synergistic effects. *Medical Vertias.* 2005; 2(2):535-542.

[96] Echeverria D, Woods JS, Heyer NJ, Rohlman D, Farin F, Li T, Garabedian CE. The association between a genetic polymorphism of coproporphyrinogen oxidase, dental mercury exposure and neurobehavioral response in humans. *Neurotoxicol Teratol.* 2006; 28(1):39-48.

[97] Woods JS, Heyer NJ, Echeverria D, Russo JE, Martin MD, Bernardo MF, Luis HS, Vaz L, Farin FM. Modification of neurobehavioral effects of mercury by a genetic polymorphism of coproporphyrinogen oxidase in children. *Neurotoxicol Teratol.* 2012; 34(5):513-21

[98] Echeverria D, Woods JS, Heyer NJ, Rohlman D, Farin FM, Li T, Garabedian CE. The association between a genetic polymorphism of coproporphyrinogen oxidase, dental mercury exposure and neurobehavioral response in humans. *Neurotoxicology and teratology.* 2006; 28(1):39-48.

[99] Godfrey ME, Wojcik DP, Krone CA. Apolipoprotein E genotyping as a potential biomarker for mercury toxicity. *Journal of Alzheimer's Disease.* 2003; 5(3):189-195.

[100] Redhe O, Pleva J. Recovery of amyotrophic lateral sclerosis and from allergy after removal of dental amalgam fillings. *Int J Risk & Safety in Med.* 1994; 4(3):229-236.

[101] Summers AO, Wireman J, Vimy MJ, Lorscheider FL, Marshall B, Levy SB, Billard L. Mercury released from dental "silver" fillings provokes an increase in mercury- and antibiotic-resistant bacteria in oral and intestinal floras of primates. *Antimicrobial agents and chemotherapy.* 1993; 37(4):825-834.

[102] Geier DA, Kern JK, Geier MR. A prospective study of prenatal mercury exposure from dental amalgams and autism severity. *Neurobiolgiae Experimentals Polish Neuroscience Society.* 2009; 69(2):189-197.

[103] Laks DR. Environmental Mercury Exposure and the Risk of Autism [white paper]. Coalition for Safe Minds; August 27, 2008.

[104] Geier DA, Kern JK, Geier MR. The biological basis of autism spectrum disorders: Understanding causation and

treatment by clinical geneticists. *Acta Neurobiol Exp (Wars).* 2010; 70(2): 209-226.

[105] Bartova J, Prochazkova J, Kratka Z, Benetkova K, Venclikova C, Sterzl I. Dental amalgam as one of the risk factors in autoimmune disease. *Neuro Endocrinol Lett.* 2003; 24(1-2):65-67.

[106] Prochazkova J, Sterzl I, Kucerkova H, Bartova J, Stejskal VDM. The beneficial effect of amalgam replacement on health in patients with autoimmunity. *Neuroendocrinology Lett.* 2004; 25(3):211-218.

[107] Sterzl I, Prochazkova J, Hrda P, Matucha P, Stejskal VD. Mercury and nickel allergy: risk factors in fatigue and autoimmunity. *Neuroendocrinol Lett.* 1999; 20(3-4):221-228.

[108] Siblerud RL. The relationship between mercury from dental amalgam and the cardiovascular system. *Science of the Total Environment.* 1990; 99(1-2):23-35.

[109] Sterzl I, Prochazkova J, Hrda P, Matucha P, Stejskal VD. Mercury and nickel allergy: risk factors in fatigue and autoimmunity. *Neuroendocrinol Lett.* 1999; 20(3-4):221-228.

[110] Stejskal I, Danersund A, Lindvall A, Hudecek R, Nordman V, Yaqob A, Mayer W, Bieger W, Lindh U. Metal-specific lymphocytes: biomarkers of sensitivity in man. *Neuroendocrinol Lett.* 1999; 20(5):289-298.

[111] Wojcik DP, Godfrey ME, Christie D, Haley BE. Mercury toxicity presenting as chronic fatigue, memory impairment and depression: diagnosis, treatment, susceptibility, and outcomes in a New Zealand general practice setting: 1994-2006. *Neuro Endocrinol Lett.* 2006; 27(4):415-423.

[112] Hanson M. Health and amalgam removal: a meta-analysis of 25 studies. *Tf-bladet Bull of the Swedish Association of Dental Mercury Patients.* Tf-bladet no. 2 2004 and SOU 2003:53 appendix 10, Sw. Dept. of Health: 204-216.

[113] Sjursen TT, Lygre GM, Dalen K, Helland V, Laegreid T, Svahn J, Lundekvam BF, Björkman L. Changes in

health complaints after removal of amalgam fillings. *Journal of Oral Rehabilitation.* 2011; 38(11): 835-848.

[114] Zamm A. Dental mercury: a factor that aggravates and induces xenobiotic intolerance. *Journal of Orthomolecular Medicine.* 1991; (6)2.

[115] Hanson M, Pleva J. The dental amalgam issue: a review. *Experientia.* 1991; 47(1):9-22.

[116] Rothwell JA, Boyd PJ. Amalgam dental fillings and hearing loss. *Int. J. Audiol.* December 2008; 47(12):770-776.

[117] Barregard L, Fabricius-Lagging E, Lundh T, Molne J, Wallin M, Olausson M, Modigh C, Sallsten G. Cadmium, mercury, and lead in kidney cortex of living kidney donors: impact of different exposure sources. *Environ Res.* 2010; 110(1):47-54.

[118] Nylander M., Friberg L, Lind B. Mercury concentrations in the human brain and kidneys in relation to exposure from dental amalgam fillings. *Swed Dent J.* 1987; 11(5):179-187.

[119] Mortada WL, Sobh MA, El-Defrawi, MM, Farahat SE. Mercury in dental restoration: is there a risk of nephrotoxity? *J Nephrol.* 2002; 15(2):171-176.

[120] Reinhardt JW. Side-effects: Mercury contribution to body burden from dental amalgam. *Adv Dent Res.* 1992; 6(1):110-3.

[121] Ely JTA, Fudenberg HH, Muirhead RJ, LaMarche MG, Krone CA, Buscher D, Stern EA. Urine Mercury in Micromercurialism: Bimodal Distribution and Diagnostic Implications. *Bulletin of Environmental Contamination and Toxicology.* 1999; 63(5):553-559.

[122] Siblerud RL. A comparison of mental health of multiple sclerosis patients with silver/mercury dental fillings and those with fillings removed. *Psychol Rep.* 1992; 70(3pt 2):1136-51.

[123] Huggins HA, Levy TE. Cerebrospinal fluid protein changes in multiple sclerosis after dental amalgam removal. *Altern Med Rev.* August 1998; 3(4):295-300.

[124] Siblerud RL, Kienholz E. Evidence that mercury from silver dental fillings may be an etiological factor in

multiple sclerosis. *The Science of the Total Environment.*
1994; 142(3):191-205.
[125] Laine J, Kalimo K, Forssell H, Happonen R.
Resolution of oral lichenoid lesions after replacement of
amalgam restorations in patients allergic to mercury
compounds. *JAMA.* 1992; 267(21):2880.
[126] Lind PO, Hurlen B, Lyberg T, Aas E. Amalgam-
related oral lichenoid reaction. *Scand J Dent Res.* 1986;
94(5):448-51.
[127] Henriksson E, Mattsson U, Håkansson J. Healing of
lichenoid reactions following removal of amalgam. A
clinical follow-up. *J Clin Periodontol.* 1995; 22(4):287-
94.
[128] Pang BK, Freeman S. Oral lichenoid lesions caused by
allergy to mercury in amalgam fillings. *Contact
Dermatitis.* 1995; 33(6):423-7.
[129] Ibbotson SH, Speight EL, Macleod RI, Smart ER,
Lawrence CM. The relevance and effect of amalgam
replacement in subjects with oral lichenoid reactions.
British Journal of Dermatology. 1996; 134(3):420-423.
[130] Dunsche A, Kastel I, Terheyden H, Springer ING,
Christopher E, Brasch J. Oral lichenoid reactions
associated with amalgam: improvement after amalgam
removal. *British Journal of Dermatology.* 2003;
148(1):70-76.
[131] Finne KAJ, Göransson K, Winckler L. Oral lichen
planus and contact allergy to mercury. *International
journal of oral surgery.* 1982; 11(4):236-239.
[132] Lundstrom, IM. Allergy and corrosion of dental
materials in patients with oral lichen planus. *Int J Oral
Surg.* 1984; 13(1):16.
[133] Mutter J. Is dental amalgam safe for humans? The
opinion of the scientific committee of the European
Commission. *Journal of Occupational Medicine and
Toxicology.* 2011; 6:2.
[134] Goldschmidt PR, Cogan RB, Taubman SB. Effects of
amalgam corrosion products on human cells. *J Period
Res.* 1976; 11(2):108-15.

[135] Ziff MF. Documented side effects of dental amalgam. *ADR.*. 1992; 6(1):131-134.
[136] Rowland AS, Baird DD, Weinberg CR, Shore DL, Shy CM, Wilcox AJ. The effect of occupational exposure to mercury vapour on the fertility of female dental assistants. *Occupat Environ Med.* 1994; 51:28-34.
[137] Sikorski R, Juszkiewicz T, Paszkowski T, Szprengier-Juszkiewicz T. Women in dental surgeries: reproductive hazards in exposure to metallic mercury. *International Archives of Occupational and Environmental Health.* 1987; 59(6): 551-557.
[138] Wojcik DP, Godfrey ME, Christie D, Haley BE. Mercury toxicity presenting as chronic fatigue, memory impairment and depression: diagnosis, treatment, susceptibility, and outcomes in a New Zealand general practice setting: 1994-2006. *Neuro Endocrinol Lett.* 2006; 27(4):415-423.
[139] Raymond LJ, Ralston NVC. Mercury: selenium interactions and health complications. *Seychelles Medical and Dental Journal.* 2004; 7(1): 72-77.
[140] Haley BE. Mercury toxicity: genetic susceptibility and synergistic effects. *Medical Vertias.* 2005; 2(2): 535-542.
[141] Haley BE. The relationship of the toxic effects of mercury to exacerbation of the medical condition classified as Alzheimer's disease. *Medical Veritas.* 2007; 4(2):1510–1524.
[142] Ingalls TH. Epidemiology, etiology, and prevention of multiple sclerosis. Hypothesis and fact. *Am. J. Forensic Med. Pathol.* 1983; 4(1):55-61.
[143] Schubert J, Riley EJ, Tyler SA. Combined effects in toxicology—a rapid systematic testing procedure: Cadmium, mercury, and lead. *Journal of Toxicology and Environmental Health*, Part A Current Issues. 1978; 4(5-6):763-776.
[144] Mata L, Sanchez L, Calvo, M. Interaction of mercury with human and bovine milk proteins. *Biosci Biotechnol Biochem.* 1997; 61(10): 1641-4.
[145] Kostial K, Rabar I, Ciganovic M, Simonovic I. Effect of milk on mercury absorption and gut retention in rats.

Bulletin of Environmental Contamination and Toxicology. 1979; 23(1): 566-571.

[146] Hursh JB, Greenwood MR, Clarkson TW, Allen J, Demuth S. The effect of ethanol on the fate of mercury inhaled by man. *JPET.* 1980; 214(3):520-527.

[147] Hanson M. 258 symptoms of mercury toxicity and 12000 mercury citations. *Mercury Bibliography (3rd edition).* Orlando, FL: Bio-Probe; 1992.

[148] von Oettingen WF. Poisoning: A Guide to Clinical Diagnosis and Treatment. *The American Journal of the Medical Sciences.* 1960; 240(3):401.

[149] International Programme on Chemical Safety. Environmental Health Criteria 1: Mercury. Geneva, Switzerland: United Nations Environment Programme and World Health Organization, 1976. http://www.inchem.org/documents/ehc/ehc/ehc001.htm.

[150] Sugita M. The biological half-time of heavy metals. The existence of a third slowest component. *Int Arch Occup Health.* 1978; 41(1):25-40.

[151] 94th U.S. Congress. H.R.11124: Medical Device Amendments. *U.S. House of Representative Bill Summary & Status.* December 11, 1975.

[152] United States Food and Drug Administration. 45 FR 85962 at 85964. *Federal Register.* December 30, 1980.

[153] United States Food and Drug Administration. 52 FR 30082. *Federal Register.* August 12, 1987.

[154] United States Food and Drug Administration. FR63(77):19799-19802. *Federal Register.* April 22, 1988.

[155] FDAnews. FDA to classify mercury fillings by summer 2009. *Daily Device Bulletin.* June 17, 2008; 5(118):1. http://www.fdanews.com/newsletter/article?issueId=11684&articleId=107723.

[156] United States Food and Drug Administration. Joint Meeting of the Dental Products Panel (CDRH) and the Peripheral and Central Nervous System Drugs Advisory Committee (CDER). September 6-7, 2006. http://www.fda.gov/AdvisoryCommittees/CommitteesMe

etingMaterials/MedicalDevices/MedicalDevicesAdvisory
Committee/DentalProductsPanel/ucm125150.htm.
[157] FDAnews. FDA to classify mercury fillings by
summer 2009. *Daily Device Bulletin.* June 17, 2008.
5(118):1.
http://www.fdanews.com/newsletter/article?issueId=1168
4&articleId=107723.
[158] United States Food and Drug Administration. Press
Announcements: FDA Issues Final Regulation on Dental
Amalgam [press release]. July 28, 2009.
http://www.fda.gov/NewsEvents/Newsroom/Pressannoun
cements/ucm173992.htm.
[159] United States Food and Drug Administration. Dental
Devices: Classification of Dental Amalgam,
Reclassification of Dental Mercury, Designation of
Special Controls for Dental Amalgam, Mercury, and
Amalgam Alloy. 2009.
http://www.fda.gov/downloads/MedicalDevices/Products
andMedicalProcedures/DentalProducts/DentalAmalgam/
UCM174024.pdf.
[160] United States Food and Drug Administration.
Addendum to the Dental Amalgam White Paper:
Response to 2006 Joint Advisory Panel Comments and
Recommendations. July 2009.
http://www.fda.gov/downloads/medicaldevices/productsa
ndmedicalprocedures/dentalproducts/dentalamalgam/ucm
173908.pdf.
[161] Associated Press. Warning issued for silver dental
fillings. *USA Today.* 6/12/2008.
[162] Love JM, Reeves RE. Petition for Reconsideration,
hereby request that the Food & Drug Administration
reconsider the classification of dental amalgam fillings
into Class II per the FDA's August 4, 2009, Final Rule
[petition]. Champion's Gate, FL: IAOMT; Sep. 3, 2009.
[163] United States of America Department of Health and
Human Services Food and Drug Administration, Center
for Devices and Radiological Health Medical Devices
Committee. Dental Products Panel [transcript].
December 15, 2010.

http://www.fda.gov/downloads/AdvisoryCommittees/Co mmitteesMeetingMaterials/MedicalDevices/MedicalDevi cesAdvisoryCommittee/DentalProductsPanel/UCM24236 3.pdf.

[164] ®andall™. Jeffrey Shuren, director of FDA's CDRH, will make end year (2011) announcement on dental amalgam. [Video Footage from FDA Townhall Meeting in California.] Uploaded January 8, 2012 by Mercury Exposure.
http://www.youtube.com/watch?v=H2t0J2_1yr0.

[165] Health Canada. *The Safety of Dental Amalgam.* Ottowa, Ontario: Minister of Health; 1996.

[166] National Institute of Dental Research. National Institute of Dental Research (NIDR) Workshop on the biocompatibility of metals in dentistry. *JADA.* 1984; 109: 169-171.

[167] American Dental Association. When your patients ask about mercury in amalgam. *JADA.* 1990; 120:395-8.

[168] American Dental Association. Dental amalgam and other restorative materials: Advisory opinion 5.A.1, American Dental Association Principles of Ethics and Code of Professional Conduct. Revised April 2002.

[169] Chirba-Martin M, Welshhans C. An uncertain risk and an uncertain future: assessing the legal implications of mercury amalgam fillings. *Health Matrix: Journal of Law-Medicine.* 2004; 14:293-324.

[170] Legal brief filed in W.H. Tolhurst vs. Johnson & Johnson Consumer Products, Inc; Engelhard Corp.; ABE Dental Inc.; The American Dental Association, et al. In the Superior Court of the State of California, In and For the Country of Santa Clara. Case No. 718228. 1995.

[171] ADA Seal of Acceptance Program & Products. American Dental Association Web site. http://www.ada.org/sealprogramproducts.aspx. Accessed August 27, 2013.

[172] Pyle, Amy. A debate on mercury in fillings. *Los Angeles Times.* October 25, 1999.
http://articles.latimes.com/1999/oct/25/news/mn-26046

[173] CBS. Is there poison in your mouth? *60 Minutes.* December 16, 1990.

[174] Sehnert KW, Jacobson G, Sullivan K. Is mercury toxicity an autoimmune disorder? *Townsend Letter for Doctors and Patients.* (1999):100-103.

[175] CBS Television Distribution. Dangerous toxins. *The Doctors.* January 3, 2013. http://www.thedoctorstv.com/main/show_synopsis/1195?section=synopsis

[176] CBS Television Distribution. Dangerous Toxins. *The Doctors.* January 3, 2013. http://www.thedoctorstv.com/videolib/init/8092

[177] Vimy MJ, Lorscheider FL. Clinical science intra-oral air mercury released from dental amalgam. *J Den Res.* 1985; 64(8):1069-71.

[178] Vimy MJ, Lorscheider FL. Serial measurements of intra-oral air mercury: estimation of daily dose from dental amalgam. *J Dent Res.* 1985; 64(8):1072-5.

[179] Hahn LJ, Kloiber R, Vimy MJ, Takahashi Y, Lorscheider F. Dental "silver" tooth fillings: a source of mercury exposure revealed by whole-body image scan and tissue analysis. *FASEB J.* 1989; 3(14):2641-2646.

[180] Harpo, Inc. Are your silver fillings making you sick? *The Dr. Oz Show.* March 28, 2013. http://www.doctoroz.com/episode/are-your-silver-fillings-making-you-sick?video=18041

[181] American Dental Association. American Dental Association Objects to the Dr. Oz show segment on dental amalgam [press release]. Chicago, Illinois American Dental Association. March 28, 2013. http://www.ada.org/8448.aspx.

[182] Dental Filling Facts. American Dental Association Web site. http://www.ada.org/sections/publicResources/pdfs/dental_fillings_facts_abstract.pdf. Accessed August 28, 2013.

[183] Begerow J. Long term urinary platinum, palladium, and gold excretion of patients after insertion of noble metal dental alloys. *Biomarkers.* 1999; 4(1):27-36.

[184] Smith DC, Williams DF. *Biocompatibility of Dental Materials, Vol III: Biocompatibility of Dental Restorative Materials*. Boca Raton, FL: CRC Press, Inc.; 1982.

[185] Wyman RJ. The Posterior Composite Resin Restoration. *Winning at Restorative Dentistry without Mercury*. Toronto, Canada: Maxplax: 1984.

[186] Richardson GM. An assessment of adult exposure and risks from components and degradation products of composite resin dental materials. *Human Ecolog Risk Assessment*. 1997; 3(4):683-697.

[187] Richardson GM, Clark KE, Williams DR. Preliminary estimates of adult exposure to bisphenol-a from dental materials, food and ambient air. *ASTM SPECIAL TECHNICAL PUBLICATION*. 1999; 1364:286-304.

[188] Richardson GM. Assessment of exposure and risks from components and degradation products of composite resin dental materials. *IAOMT*. 1996.

[189] Richardson GM. Mercury exposure and risks from dental amalgam in Canada: The Canadian Health Measures Survey 2007-2009. *Human and Ecological Risk Assessment: An International Journal*. 2012.

[190] McCracken MS, Gordan VV, Litaker MS, Funkhouser E, Fellows JL, Shamp DG, Qvist V, Meral JS, Gilbert GH. A 24-month evaluation of amalgam and resin-based composite restorations Findings from The National Dental Practice-Based Research Network. *The Journal of the American Dental Association*. 2013; 144(6):583-593.

[191] Laccabue M, Ahlf RL, Simecek JW. Frequency of Restoration Replacement in Posterior Teeth for US Navy and Marine Corps Personnel. *Operative dentistry*. 2013.

[192] Heintze SD, Rousson V. Clinical effectiveness of direct Class II restorations—a meta-analysis. *J Adhes Dent*. 2012; 14(5):407-431.

[193] Davidovich E, Weiss E, Fuks AB, Beyth N. Surface antibacterial properties of glass ionomer cements used in atraumatic restorative treatment. *The Journal of the American Dental Association*. 2007; 138(10): 1347.

[194] Lopez N, Simpser-Rafalin S, Berthold P. Atraumatic restorative treatment for prevention and treatment of

caries in an underserved community. *American journal of public health.* 2005; 95(8): 1338-1339.

[195] World Health Organization. Future Use of Materials for Dental Restoration: Report of the Meeting Convened at WHO HQ, Geneva, Switzerland. Geneva, Switzerland: WHO, November 2009.

[196] Heintze SD, Rousson V. Clinical effectiveness of direct Class II restorations—a meta-analysis. *J Adhes Dent.* 2012; 14(5):407-431.

[197] Lindqvist B, Mörnstad H. Effects of removing amalgam fillings from patients with diseases affecting the immune system. *Medical Science Research.* May 1996; 24(5):355-356.

[198] Siblerud RL. A comparison of mental health of multiple sclerosis patients with silver/mercury dental fillings and those with fillings removed. *Psychol Rep.* 1992; 70(3pt 2):1136-51.

[199] Huggins HA, Levy TE. Cerebrospinal fluid protein changes in multiple sclerosis after dental amalgam removal. *Altern Med Rev.* 1998; 3(4):295-300.

[200] Siblerud RL, Kienholz E. Evidence that mercury from silver dental fillings may be an etiological factor in multiple sclerosis. *The Science of the Total Environment.* 1994; 142(3):191-205.

[201] Redhe O, Pleva J. Recovery of amyotrophic lateral sclerosis and from allergy after removal of dental amalgam fillings. *Int J Risk & Safety in Med.* 1994; 4(3):229-236.

[202] Prochazkova J, Sterzl I, Kucerkova H, Bartova J, Stejskal VDM. The beneficial effect of amalgam replacement on health in patients with autoimmunity. *Neuroendocrinology Lett.* 2004; 25(3):211-218.

[203] Zamm AV. Candida albicans therapy. Is there ever an end to it? Dental mercury removal: an effective adjunct. *J. Orthomol. Med.* 1986; 1(4): 261-266.

[204] Sjursen TT, Lygre GM, Dalen K, Helland V, Laegreid T, Svahn J, Lundekvam BF, Björkman L. Changes in health complaints after removal of amalgam fillings. *Journal of Oral Rehabilitation.* 2011; 38(11):835-848.

87

[205] Wojcik DP, Godfrey ME, Christie D, Haley BE. Mercury toxicity presenting as chronic fatigue, memory impairment and depression: diagnosis, treatment, susceptibility, and outcomes in a New Zealand general practice setting: 1994-2006. *Neuro Endocrinol Lett.* 2006; 27(4): 415-423.

[206] Laine J, Kalimo K, Forssell H, Happonen R. Resolution of oral lichenoid lesions after replacement of amalgam restorations in patients allergic to mercury compounds. *JAMA.* 1992; 267(21):2880.

[207] Fleming M and Janosky J. The Economics of Dental Amalgam Regulation. Report Submitted for Review and Publication to "Public Health Reports. Available online at http://iaomt.guiadmin.com/wp-content/uploads/The-Economics-of-Dental-Amalgam-Regulation.pdf.

[208] Maryniuk GA. In search of treatment longevity - A 30 year perspective. *JADA.* 1984; 109(5):739-744.

[209] Walls AWG, Wallwork MA, Holland IS, and Murray JJ. The longevity of occlusal amalgam restorations in first permanent molars of child patients. *Br. Dent J.* 1985; 158(4):133-136.

[210] Rom WN, Ed. Environmental and Occupational Medicine. Boston: Little, Brown, and Co. 1983:461.

[211] Sears ME, Kerr KJ, Bray RI. Arsenic, cadmium, lead, and mercury in sweat: a systematic review. *Journal of environmental and public health.* 2012.

[212] Stejskal VDM, Cederbrant K, Lindvall A, Forsbeck M. MELISA—an *in vitro* tool for the study of metal allergy. *Toxicology in vitro.* 1994; 8(5):991-1000.

[213] ADA Council on Scientific Affairs; ADA Council on Dental Benefit Porgrams. Statement on posterior Resin based composites. *JADA.* 1998; 129(11):1627-8

[214] McGrath K. A Toxic Mouthful: the Misalignment of Dental Mercury Regulations. *B.C.J.L. & Soc. Just.* 2013; 33(2):347. http://lawdigitalcommons.bc.edu/jlsj/vol33/iss2/4

[215] United Nations Environment Programme. Minamata Convention on Mercury. Geneva, Switzerland: Text agreed upon in UNEP(DTIE)/Hg/INC.5/3; January 13-19, 2013.
http://www.mercuryconvention.org/Portals/11/documents/conventionText/Minamata%20Convention%20on%20Mercury_e.pdf

[216] Informed Consent. American Medical Association Web site. http://www.ama-assn.org/ama/pub/physician-resources/legal-topics/patient-physician-relationship-topics/informed-consent.page. Accessed August 28, 2013.

[217] Dental Board of California. The Facts about Fillings [fact sheet]. Sacramento, CA: California Department of Consumer Affairs; 5/04.
http://www.dbc.ca.gov/formspubs/pub_dmfs_english_webview.pdf

[218] State of Connecticut Department of Environmental Protection. Fillings: The Choices You Have: Mercury Amalgam and Other Filling Materials [brochure]. Hartford, CT: DEP; May 2011.
http://www.ct.gov/dep/lib/dep/mercury/gen_info/fillings_brochure.pdf.

[219] Maine Bureau of Health. Filling Materials [brochure]. Augusta, ME: Bureau of Health, 2002.
http://www.vce.org/mercury/Maine_AmalBrochFinal2.pdf.

[220] Advisory Committee on Mercury Pollution. Dental Amalgam Fillings: Environmental and Health Facts for Dental Patients [brochure]. Waterbury, Vermont: Mercury Education and Reduction Campaign.
http://www.mercvt.org/PDF/DentalAmalgamFactSheet.pdf. Accessed August 22, 2013.

NOTES

NOTES

NOTES